THE COMPLETE GUIDE TO THE
PILATES METHOD

from lower back pain to muscle conditioning

by

Allan Menezes
BAdmin.MSc.GInstM.MPIA.

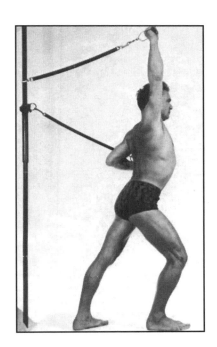

"Physical fitness is the first prerequisite of happiness" - J.H.Pilates. (1880 -1967)

Ahead in Marketing - Sydney

ACKNOWLEDGEMENTS

My thanks go to all my staff and franchisees (Simon and Vanessa Wood of Body Control Studios Parramatta, Sydney and Sefulu Calvert of Body Control Studios Wellington, New Zealand) who have been extremely patient while this book has been in various stages of its development. For the input they have provided and in the expansion of the Body Control Pilates Studios to the largest organization of its kind in the world. To my father for handing me that voucher that changed my life, and started an industry in Australia. To my mother who, without my knowing it at the time, gave me my best motivation. To all my clients, past and present, who have all contributed towards the refinement of the routines by allowing me over the years to test new exercises and perfect old ones. Most importantly, my thanks and appreciation go to my wife, Sonja, who has displayed the ultimate in patience and encouragement through many frustrating moments in this book's long journey to its conclusion. What a source of determination, perseverance and inspiration!

The author also wishes to thank Daniel Mathieu for the illustrations, KC for the great photographs, and Vanessa Wood, Simon Wood and Jennifer Scott for modelling for the photos.

The Complete Guide to the Pilates Method - from lower back pain to muscle conditioning.

First published in Australia in 1998 by Ahead in Marketing.
Second printing 2000 by Pilates Institute of Australasia Pty Ltd.

National Library of Australia
Cataloguing-in-Publication data

Menezes, A. S. (Allan S.)

    ISBN 0-646-35767-0

Pilates Method, Pilates
    i)   Back Pain
    ii)   Muscle Conditioning
    iii)   Stretching

Published by Pilates Institute of Australasia
P.O. Box 1046, North Sydney
New South Wales 2059 Australia
Tel +61 2 9267 8223
Fax +61 2 9267 8226
Internet www.pilates.net

Contrology® and Reformer® are registered trademarks licensed to the Pilates Institute of Austalasia Pty Ltd.

Body Control Pilates™ is a trademark of Body Control Australia Pty Ltd and is not associated with any other organisation outside Australasia.

Cover - background - Joseph Pilates with the Pedi-Pul.
      - photos - Simon Wood, Vanessa Wood, Allan Menezes.

Design and layout in Australia by Lithium Innovation Pty Ltd (02) 9211 9596.
Printed in Australia by Australian Print Group.

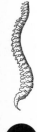

To my wife, Sonja

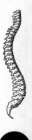

CONTENTS

PAGE

FORWARD... 8
BIOGRAPHY... 9
PREFACE.. 10
INTRODUCTION 11

CHAPTER 1

LIFE'S LIKE THAT.. 14
LOOKING FORWARD TO THE FUTURE... 14
ESTABLISHING FAULTY PATTERNS OF MOVEMENT.................................. 15
LOADING THE BODY AND THE STRETCH FACTOR.................................... 17
THE IMPORTANCE OF LEVERS.. 18
YOU CAN!.. 20

CHAPTER 2

MIND OVER MATTER... 24
THE MENTAL FACTOR... 25
DEVELOPING A "THINKING BODY".. 26
THE SKELETON AND VERTEBRAL COLUMN... 27
THE MAJOR MUSCLES... 28
THE 8 PRINCIPLES OF THE PILATES METHOD.. 29
        1. CONCENTRATION.. 30
        2. CENTERING.. 30
        3. BREATHING.. 33
        4. CONTROL... 36
        5. PRECISION... 37
        6. FLOWING MOVEMENT.. 37
        7. ISOLATION... 38
        8. ROUTINE... 39

CHAPTER 3

POSTURE

BODY TYPES & FACTORS INFLUENCING POSTURE..................................... 42
TRIPOD & POSTURAL ASSESSMENT.. 43
MUSCLE IMBALANCES... 44
IDENTIFYING PAIN... 46
OVERSTRETCHING, OVERWORKING, OVERDOING IT. PAIN!!!................. 48
BODY POSTURE FOR BETTER EXERCISING... 49
ESTABLISHING A PATTERN FOR MUSCULAR CONTROL............................ 50
THE FUNDAMENTALS OF BODY AWARENESS.. 54
FOOT POSITIONS... 55
THE CENTRE... 56

CONTENTS

CHAPTER 4 PAGE

STRETCH, STRENGTHEN AND RELIEF 61

STRETCHING AND FLEXIBILITY 62
WARMING UP 62
POINTERS FOR SAFE EXERCISING 63
THE STRUCTURE OF THE EXERCISE PROGRAM 64

CHAPTER 5

THE COMPLETE PROGRAMS 67

Exercise#
1	REST POSITION	69

THE WARM UP

2	STANDING SPINE ROLL	70
3/4/5/6/7	START STRETCHES	71
8-1	CALF STRETCH	74
8-2	ALTERNATING CALF STRETCH	75
9-1	HAMSTRINGS - SUPINE	76
9-2	HAMSTRINGS - STANDING	77
10	HAMSTRINGS - SEATED	77
11	QUAD STRETCH - I PRONE	78
12	QUAD STRETCH - II STANDING	79
13	QUAD STRETCH - III KNEELING	80

BASIC ROUTINE FOR LOWER BACK PAIN AND WEAK ABDOMINALS

14	ONE LEG LIFTS - SUPINE	81
15	SLIDING LEG	82
	SUPINE REST POSITION & CUSHION POSITION	83
16	PREPARATION I - CUSHION	84
17	PREPARATION II	85
18	HUNDREDS - BASIC	86
19	HUNDREDS - BEST ANGLE & PERCUSSION BREATHING	87
20	SINGLE LEG STRETCH	88
21	DOUBLE LEG STRETCH - BASIC	89
22	SINGLE LEG CIRCLES	90
23	SIDE TO SIDE	91
24	STOMACH STRETCHES	92
25	PERFECT ABDOMINAL CURL	93
26-I	ANKLE WEIGHTS - STRAIGHT LEG	94
26-II	ANKLE WEIGHTS - INNER THIGH	95
26-III	ANKLE WEIGHTS - OUTER THIGH FLEXION	96
27	BACK OF THIGHS - BUTTOCKS	97
28	ARM WEIGHTS - PREPARATION	98
28-1	ARM WEIGHTS - OPENINGS	99
28-2	- ALTERNATING	99
28-3	- OVERHEAD	100
28-4	- CIRCLES	100
29-1	ARM SWINGS - ALTERNATING	101
29-2	ARM SWINGS - CHEST EXPANSION	102
30	POLE	103

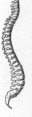

INTERMEDIATE ROUTINE
PAGE

31	HUNDREDS ALTERNATING	104
32	CO-ORDINATION	105
33	ROLL-UP	106
	THE PSOAS & IT'S EFFECT ON THE BACK	107
34	ROLL OVER	108
35	SINGLE LEG CIRCLE	109
36	DOUBLE LEG STRETCH & VARIATIONS	110
37	ROLLING	112
38	SINGLE LEG STRETCH (CRISS CROSS)	113
39	STOMACH STRETCHES - ALTERNATING ARMS & LEGS	114
40	SINGLE LEG KICK	115
41	DOUBLE LEG KICK	116
42	SWANDIVE I	117
42-I	SWANDIVE II	118
43	SWIMMING	118
44	SPINE ROTATION / TWIST	119
45	SPINE STRETCH	120
46	OPEN LEG ROCKER	121
47	CORKSCREW BASIC	122
47-I	CORKSCREW INTERMEDIATE	122
47-II	CORKSCREW ADVANCED	123
48	SAW...	124
49	SIDE KICK I	125
50	SIDE LEG LIFTS I & II	126
51	PELVIC CURL	127
52	PELVIC LIFT	128
53-I	TEASER I	129
53-II	TEASER II	130
53-III	TEASER III	131
54	LEG PULL FRONT	132
55	LEG PULLS BACK	133
56	SIDE KICK II	134
57	BOOMERANG	135
58	SEAL	136
59	CONTROL BALANCE	137

ADVANCED ROUTINE

60	HUNDREDS - LOWER & RAISE	138
61	ROLL OVER WITH BENT LEGS	139
62	PENDULUM	140
63	NECK PULL	141
64	JACKNIFE	142
65	SCISSORS	143
66	BICYCLE	144
67	SHOULDER BRIDGE	145
68	CAN CAN	146
68-I	CAN CAN EXTENSION	147
69	HIP CIRCLES	148
70	HELICOPTER HUNDREDS	149
71	LYING TORSO STRETCH	150
72	STANDING SIDE STRETCHES	151
73	CAT STRETCH	152

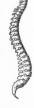

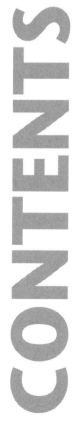

CONTENTS

74   ROCKING.. 153
75-I   TWIST I.. 154
75-II   TWIST II... 155

FURTHER SPECIFIC EXERCISES

76   OBLIQUE CURLS.. 156
77   WRIST & FOREARM STRENGTHENER........................... 157
78   NECK STRETCHES... 158
79   SEATED SPINE ROTATION.. 159
80   CUSHION SQUEEZE... 160

IsoToner ™ ROUTINE

IT1   POINTING THE FOOT.. 161
IT2   POINTING THE TOES.. 161
IT3   DORSI FLEXION OF THE ANKLE................................... 161
IT4   EVERSION OF THE ANKLE.. 161
IT5   INVERSION OF THE METATARSAL JOINT....................... 162
IT6   ADDUCTION OF THE INNER THIGH.............................. 162
IT7   FLEXION AND EXTENSION OF THE LEG.......................... 162
IT8   HYPEREXTENSION TO EXTENSION............................... 162
IT9   FLEXION AND EXTENSION ON THE BACK........................ 162
IT10   PRONE HYPEREXTENSION TO EXTENSION..................... 163
IT11   BICEPS.. 163
IT12   TRICEPS.. 163
IT13   PECTORALS (CHEST).. 163
IT14   PECTORALS AND DELTOIDS.. 163
IT15   LATISSIMUS DORSI.. 163
IT16   BACK.. 164
IT17   OVERHEAD... 164
IT18   SIDE STRETCH.. 164

CHAPTER 6

MOVE YOURSELF OUT OF PAIN.. 166
THE CONDITIONS AND THE ROUTINES WHICH BRING RELIEF............ 168
ANKLES AND FEET... 168
THE KNEE... 168
THE HIP JOINT... 168
THE BACK... 169
THE SHOULDERS.. 171
THE CHALLENGE.. 172

CONCLUSION

CONCLUSION.. 175

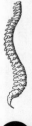

FORWARD

Finally this book has arrived!

I recommend to everyone in search of a leaner, stronger, more flexible body to use this manual as the key component in achieving their goals.

"The Complete Guide to the Pilates Method" contains the most comprehensive instruction on the Pilates Method to date. The combination of precise detail and illustrations provides a clear and easy resource for this renowned exercise program.

Those who can benefit from this book range from triathletes to ballet dancers, from new mothers to those who suffer from lower back pain.

The section on the "B-Line" I found not only interesting, but also of great assistance to abdominal bracing applied in a different, effective style. The detail is also relevant to those wishing to study the Pilates Method with a view to applying its teachings.

This is an inspiration to those who have attempted other exercise programs and found them wanting. With this guide you will not only discover your own body, you will understand it and apply a process to it that delivers results.

Allan has contributed tremendously to the emergence of the Pilates Method as its pioneer in Australia. This book further consolidates his position as the leading Pilates practitioner in the country. Allan's willingness to share his specific insights to his teaching of the Pilates Method is to be congratulated.

Make the most of this book - it works!

Peter Green DO
Course Co-ordinator of Osteopathy
University of Western Sydney
Sydney
Australia

FORWARD

BIOGRAPHY

ALLAN MENEZES is the founder and owner of Body Control Australia, and the founder of the Pilates Institute of Australasia.

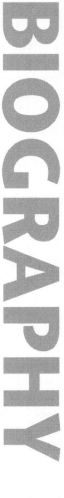

Allan suffered a debilitating back injury in a rugby accident while at university, which hospitalised him and virtually ended his athletic career. After two years of chronic lower back pain, he attended a Pilates studio in London in 1982. The daily visits cured his back problem. This convinced him that a huge, untapped market existed for the application of this method - BACK PAIN - and he changed careers to become an instructor with the Alan Herdman Studios. Allan introduced the Pilates Method to Australia in November 1986, and now runs three studios in Sydney as well as franchises in Sydney and Wellington, New Zealand.

Menezes has a very strong history of participation in sports such as tennis, swimming, squash, volleyball, basketball, cricket, track and field, karate, rugby union, gridiron, cross-country running, skiing, weight-training, etc. In many of these sports he has represented his school, college and university, and set many records in the track and field. At college and university level he was volleyball, basketball and rugby captain and, of course, has his fair share of injuries.

Allan received his Pilates Teacher Trainer Certification from the former Institute for the Pilates Method in Sante Fe, New Mexico in 1992. He is also a former Advisory Board Member of the Institute.

In 1996 Allan founded the Pilates Institute of Australasia to ensure that quality training and consistently high standards in Pilates training were established. The Institute's workshops are accredited by the Australian Fitness Accreditation Council (AFAC), the Chiropractors Education Committee and the Australian Natural Therapies Association (ANTA).

He has lectured internationally on the Pilates Method, and also conducts workshops for the general public as well as for physiotherapists, medical practitioners and other rehabilitation specialists.

The Body Control Pilates Studios and the Pilates Institute have been featured regularly in most of the country's major magazines and newspapers. There have also been several television and radio interviews, and a feature in Entrepreneur International Magazine (USA) in 1998.

Allan lives in Sydney with his wife, Sonja, and daughters, Jessica and Analiese.

PREFACE

This book was necessary. It was created by the need to have a more up to date version of an exercise routine developed by Josef Pilates in the early 1920s. It is well accepted, even by Joe Pilates himself, that he was fifty years ahead of his time. Many of his advocates, who respect and honour his work, also feel that if Joe were alive today, he would have progressed much of his work 'to the next level'.

His outstanding insights into the movement of the human body came naturally to him. Many advanced instructors throughout the world, who have been followers of the method for many years, have developed those same insights. By utilising Joe's techniques, variations have been developed which in many cases are improvements on the original. I have presented here, as much as possible, the original versions of the method and variations that have been developed over time, including routines to cater for those with lower back pain.

This book really began when I first discovered Pilates in London in 1982. After several months I moved on to the Alan Herdman Studios where I learned some of the best grounding in the Method I have ever encountered. Alan is one of the Master Teachers of the Method. Two years previously, while studying for a business degree at university, I had injured my back in a rugby game.

The injury was so severe that I lay in a hospital bed for ten days and only allowed liquids for nourishment. The diagnosis at the time was a slipped disc. X-rays showed no abnormalities and no scans were taken. My own conclusion is that the muscles on the left of the spinal column had been so badly ruptured that any pressure on that side caused extreme pain in the lower back. For the following two years I attended almost every different practitioner I could think of in the hope of alleviating the pain.

Then in London, my father handed me an introductory voucher for this 'new' method that was being taught in a small, basement studio. Little did I know that the method was 70 years new! After attending classes every day for six weeks my back pain disappeared! Regular sessions followed for the next two to three years and the back pain has not returned to this day. I was an instant convert. The one drawback was that my original instructors had very little anatomical or athletic knowledge. They could not explain the whys and wherefores of a movement and its application to me as an (ex) athlete.

I then devised my own routines for improving my squash, volleyball, etc. and programs for other fitness enthusiasts. These proved to be popular as more exertion was required and the routines became hard work. (Many years later I discovered, from a CAT scan, that I had actually herniated my disc at L4/L5! I had been living pain free owing to the regular daily workout to which I had committed myself in my Pilates training.)

It was in 1986 that I then established the first Pilates studio in the Southern Hemisphere with the Body Control Pilates Studios in Sydney. (There is no connection with any other studios with the same, or similar, names outside Australia and New Zealand). In 1994, after setting up 2 more studios, I established the first true franchise of a Pilates studio and in 1996 the Pilates Institute of Australasia was founded. This Institute was created to cater for the growing demand for quality training and to provide accredited workshops and courses in the Pilates Method.

As the demand for Pilates continues to grow, I feel this will be an invaluable text for those wishing to reduce those niggling aches and pains. It is also important for those wishing to become familiar with the basics steps in sensible body maintenance and even those embarking on a career in the growing Pilates industry. It is a basis for, not only perfection in movement, but also a requirement for the next step into exercising for physical rehabilitation. I hope that you will learn and benefit from the ideas contained here for a better body, a healthier mind and limitless energy.

DISCLAIMER

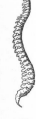

Please consult your doctor or practitioner before commencing any new exercise regime Any application of the exercises or suggestions contained in this book are undertaken by the reader after having sought the appropriate advice. The author and publisher of this book and their employers are not liable or responsible for any damage or injury caused directly or indirectly by the information contained herein.

The Complete Guide to the Pilates Method

INTRODUCTION

The basis of the Pilates Method is the art of Contrology® (a word coined by Pilates himself). "It is the conscious control of all muscular movements in the body. It is the correct utilization and application of the leverage principles afforded by the bones comprising the skeletal framework of the body, a complete knowledge of the mechanism of the body, and a full understanding of the principles of equilibrium and gravity as applied to the movements of the body in motion, at rest and in sleep." - J.Pilates

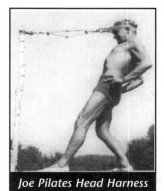
Joe Pilates Head Harness

Josef Humbertus Pilates was born in 1880 near Dusseldorf, Germany. He grew up suffering rickets, asthma and rheumatic fever. Like so many who have gone on to excel in the area of physical achievement and innovation, Pilates became obsessed with the frailties of the body and was determined to overcome his own afflictions. As a teenager, he became skilled in gymnastics, skiing and skin-diving. His determination and application to work his body to better health meant that, at 14, he was not only studying the musculature of the body, he was also able to pose for anatomical drawings. His studies also included Eastern forms of exercise and, merging these with his Western physical studies, the Pilates Method was born. Pilates named this method Contrology.

In 1912 Joe went to England where he became a boxer, circus performer and a self-defence instructor. When World War I erupted he was incarcerated in Lancaster and on the Isle of Man, with other German nationals, as 'enemy aliens'. During this time, many of his compatriots, following his exercise regime, emerged unscathed by an influenza epidemic that had swept the nation killing thousands.

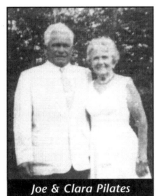
Joe & Clara Pilates

Those in the camp, who were disabled by other wartime diseases, soon discovered the benefits of having Joe within their midst. His innovative style helped him devise the forerunner of today's equipment. Joe would remove the bedsprings from beneath the beds and attach them to the walls above the patients' bed. In this manner they were able to exercise while lying down. Not only could his 'patients' remain stable, despite whatever injuries they may have had, they were also able to mobilise themselves, strengthen their muscles and emerge fitter and healthier than if these simple procedures were not available to them. When the Great War ended, Pilates returned to Germany where he continued to develop his work.

In 1926 Joe decided to emigrate to the United States, when he felt his ideals did not match those of the New German Army. On the journey across the Atlantic, he met Clara, a nurse, who was to become his wife. 'We talked so much about health and the need to keep the body healthy, we decided to open a physical fitness studio,' said Clara. This was when his teachings became known to the dance world. Rudolf von Laban, the founder of Labanotation, incorporated several of Joe's principles into his teaching, as, later, did Hanya Holm, Martha Graham, George Balanchine and others.

Josef Pilates explained his own definition of fitness in 1945 as: 'The attainment and maintenance of a uniformly developed body with a sound mind fully capable of naturally, easily and satisfactorily performing our many and varied daily tasks with spontaneous zest and pleasure.'

Pilates had a firm belief that he was fifty years ahead of his time. Even today, although the original method has changed as it has spread across the globe, the basic principles incorporated in the method still hold true.

Originally the Pilates Method was embraced by the dance world with great fervour. Consequently, more than 80% of studios and method teachers around the world are from a dance background. The movements, being fluid in nature and lengthening in structure, still have a 'balletic' appearance to them.

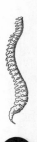

To apply the method to a tennis player, rugby fullback or baseball pitcher would be extremely difficult without having played that sport or having a strong knowledge of athletic movement. As dance is, generally, of an equal physical demand on both sides of the body, a dance-based instructor is ideal to be trained in these other disciplines.

As the method expands to those areas outside the dance world, I have attempted to structure this book so that it can be used by anyone for basic movements of the method, and as a definitive guide to those wishing to follow a sensible program that does produce results.

The principles have been refined over the years with more in-depth explanation of the muscles being used and the benefits of each exercise. Even the simplest of the routines gently leads you to more physical challenges, improved mental focus and increased health benefits.

A recent report by the Surgeon General in the United States, after decades of research on the effects of physical activity and health, reported that regular physical activity:

- reduces the risk of dying prematurely
- reduces the risk of dying from heart disease
- reduces the risk of developing diabetes
- reduces the risk of developing high blood pressure
- helps reduce blood pressure in people who already have high blood pressure
- reduces the risk of developing colon cancer
- reduces feelings of depression and anxiety
- helps weight control
- helps the aged become stronger and more mobile
- improves psychological well-being.

Gyms, with their fast circuit classes and heavy weight machines, work on the muscles groups that are already strong. Consequently, the strong muscle groups remain strong (and can get bulkier) and the weaker ones remain weak or marginally stronger at best.

The Pilates Method works from within the body towards the exterior surfaces; unlike a gym where, the work is from the outside and works towards the inside. With gym routines, once one stops, the results do not last long and the body becomes 'out of shape' fairly fast. Initially, with the Pilates Method, results may not be immediate. But, long term, the benefits will become obvious. When you stop the method for a time, the results still stay with you. And restarting, even after a two-year break, it will feel as if you had only stopped yesterday.

By working from 'the inside out' you develop a greater understanding of the body. Smaller muscle groups come into use and you begin to discover muscles that you thought you never had or, what you once thought was fat actually has a 'hidden' muscle there! Further, it develops a control that is capable of being achieved in the simplest of movements; from walking up a flight of stairs to the most 'complex', such as lifting an awkward load from a difficult position without straining the back, shoulders or other muscles.

The aim of the method is to produce:

1. Fluidity and awareness of movement,
2. Mental focus and control over these movements without the need to concentrate on them,
3. A body that 'thinks' for itself,
4. A healthy body both inside and out.

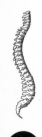

CHAPTER 1

*"Man should bear in mind and ponder over the Greek admonition
- not too much, not too little" - J.Pilates*

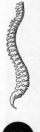

CHAPTER 1

LIFE'S LIKE THAT

Have you ever wished for MORE mental and physical stamina for playing longer with the children or grandchildren, completing the daily household duties or even playing that extra game of tennis without becoming over fatigued? Have you ever wished for MORE energy at the end of each day, rather than feeling drained? Have you ever wondered why people accept the back pain with which they live?

Why do we act and move the way we do? Why do we sometimes feel the same aches and pains as our parents do? Why do we develop new ones that our parents did not have? Will we acquire the same maladies with which elderly people become afflicted?

To a great extent, the answer to much of this can be found in our current lifestyle. The fast pace, our eating habits, the effects of the greenhouse gases and so on. The continuation of this type of lifestyle can lead to mental and physical stress, thereby causing the body to 'breakdown' under the pressure. This pressure then manifests itself in several forms. These can range from mild allergies to severe and chronic aches and pains, various types of injuries and these stresses can even lead to the breakdown of our personal relationships.

This can have a lasting effect on our normal behaviour pattern. That is why we feel the urge to 'get away from it all'. To escape to the mountains or the coast, to a quieter, more tranquil environment where we can 'be ourselves'. But at the end of the getaway we have to face it all over again the next week. How are we supposed to cope with these pressures of life? How do we control our bodies so that they do not give way on us? Ultimately, how do we live longer, happier, healthier lives?

LOOKING FORWARD TO THE FUTURE.

We can usually do very little about our 'inherited conditions'. We cannot change the colour of our eyes or the tone of our skin. As we develop, we then begin to learn from those around us - our parents, our teachers, our peers and those with whom we come into contact. As we learn from these experiences, whether good or bad, we tend to use them as reference points in our lives. We develop a mindset of what our abilities and capabilities are, by what we are told we can and cannot do.

As children we are influenced by the environment in which we live. We study at school and learn from our parents certain 'ingrained' values, morals and lifestyle patterns that become programmed into our influential behaviour grid. As we see our parents', teachers' and peers' behaviour, we tend to copy them as part of our own and develop habitual patterns similar to theirs. As we see the behaviour of our peers we may want to go with what is 'cool', such as smoking. This would greatly affect our future health patterns.

As school children, we would have a tendency to carry a heavy bag full of school books, predominantly over one shoulder. The effect of this is the strong possibility of developing a scoliosis of the spine. As we continue to follow this pattern, as our body physically develops and grows, something else can affect us later in life, such as back pain.

Various mental and emotional beliefs that we adhere to through our lives may then become patterns and can manifest themselves in physical ways. Because of our lack of self-esteem or our fear of 'adventure', our image of ourselves becomes set. We tend to do things in certain ways and in certain patterns. We shop at the same supermarket, we go to the same holiday destinations, we walk in a fixed gait, and we move and feed our bodies in an habitual way. We do make the occasional attempt to improve ourselves by going on healthy diets or making the determined commitment to go to the gym three times a week for the rest of our lives!

As we do attempt to achieve more and improve ourselves, we find a constant need to refine what we are doing and the way in which we do it. To accomplish these higher goals, whether in the workplace or in our personal relationships, our physical and mental makeup bears the brunt of the enforced new routine. In order to handle difficult situations on a day to day basis with the changes we undertake, we require our bodies to provide us with more mental and physical support and energy. The adage of 'healthy body, healthy mind' is truer today than it has ever been. Even truer still is one of Joe Pilates' favourite quotes, that of the German philosopher, Schiller, 'It is the mind which controls the body'.

Establishing faulty patterns of movement

Our workplace environment has become more sedentary and our leisure time has followed suit. Children now spend more time in front of the television than ever before and these habits tend to follow into adulthood. The era of the 'couch potato' has been upon us and we have not noticed it until almost too late. The immobility that results from not using our bodies as we once did before we became bipedal, has not only restricted our movements in our joints but has also placed our bodies and muscles in an 'unbalanced configuration' (Fig.1).

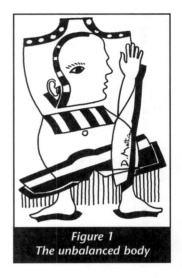

Figure 1
The unbalanced body

What this means is that we tend to favour one group of muscles more than another when we perform most of our day to day activities, eg. we would throw or kick a ball with the same arm or leg, women would tend to hold a baby on predominantly the same hip, we would hold a telephone to one ear with the same hunched shoulder, etc. These one-sided actions cause imbalances in the body. Even the way we walk with an unnoticeable longer stride in one leg can unbalance our musculo-skeletal structures and can lead to back pain and even migraines!

These continuous, repetitive movements over a period of time become 'set' in the memory of the muscle and may never affect us until one day we attempt a different movement. These set movements, or engrams as they are known, stay with us for many years. If we have not ridden a bicycle for many years we are still capable of doing so without falling off as often as we did when we were children. These engrams have also set a neuromuscular pattern in our brain so certain movements become habitual. The problems occur when we change the habit.

This, then, becomes our physical 'safety zone'. Even if we know we move in a certain, ungainly way (usually because it's been pointed out to us, not because we have noticed it ourselves), we feel it is 'normal'.

For example, walking with slight knock-knees. The movement is not grossly distorted. It is, however, noticeable to others. The movement to the person seems 'normal', the gait feels just a fast and fluid in execution as anyone else's; but it is not how 90% of the population walk! If the gait is to be corrected, the inherent pattern of movement requires change. Even though there may have been no physical discomfort, change would be required if it inhibits progress; in this case, such as speed for a 100-meter race, or as a model to walk down a catwalk.

In most cases this realignment of the body's 'abnormal' position to what is normal, requires a re-education of the musculature (assuming there are no structural (skeletal) problems).

Similar muscular 'pulls' occur in many of our everyday movements; women who wear high heels would walk with a forward tilt, this is corrected by leaning backwards. The result is a forward tilt of the pelvis and the compensation of the backward lean would tend to arch and tighten the lower back.

Case study:

Patient A stands normally and outwardly appears not to have any structural problems.
However, Patient A cannot touch his toes from a standing position, even after extensive stretching and exercise. Hamstring stretches on the individual legs are without problems and quite flexible; the lower back is moderately tight.

A decision was made to invert the client. Upon relaxing in an inverted position, Patient A was found to have a marked rotation of the spine not evident in the normal standing position. After a series of appropriate exercises to counter the imbalance Patient A was easily able to touch his toes.

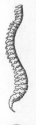

In the above case study we see that, without our knowledge, our body will align itself according to a frame of reference. This frame of reference being a 'squaring' of the torso when standing. Visual images of what is straight and correct alignment are imprinted in our subconscious from what we see around us. We then stand accordingly, even if this is not our 'natural' position (Fig.2).

Children who experience growth spurts and outgrow their peers tend to walk with stooped shoulders, so as not to bring attention to themselves when they are head and shoulders above the rest. This action tightens the pectoral group of muscles in the chest resulting in rounded shoulders or stooped posture. The neck may need to be lengthened to appear more upright. If the shoulders are not corrected at the same time, a greater arch than normal in the neck can occur with its associated problems of neck pain, headaches and even back pain. In addition, the muscles in the middle of the back, between the shoulder blades (the rhomboids), would need strengthening and the chest muscles lengthening.

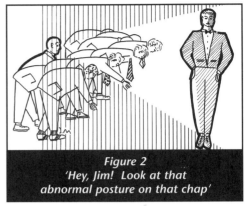

Figure 2
'Hey, Jim! Look at that abnormal posture on that chap'

In the example of the woman in high heels, various gravitational forces may tend to tighten the muscles on either side of the spine to such an extent that, even when standing on a flat surface, there is discomfort in the back. This may be a result of tight calves, leading to tight quadriceps, leading to tight psoas muscles, leading to tight lower back muscles. Other factors may also be involved, such as lack of exercise or weak abdominals, which would also influence the condition (Fig.3).

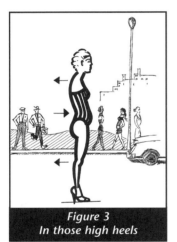

Figure 3
In those high heels

These instances tend not to be of great concern if they do not cause discomfort. However, the many years of repeating the same action tends to 'set' the muscle into what then becomes its 'normal' pattern.

Tightness in one group of muscles invariably indicates a weakness in another, usually opposite, group of muscles. In the high heel example above, the weak areas that would be identified would be the abdominals. However, strengthening the abdominals is not the total solution to the condition. Stretching and lengthening the tight muscles is also of great importance in order to alleviate the problem. Control of these muscles on a continual basis is important. If the lower back is arched due to weak abdominals, then concentration is required to 'pull' these in, even when standing at a bus stop. To remind the muscles to do the right thing will eventually lead to a more comfortable posture. It is easier to let the body not think for itself, than it is to remind it what to do for ten seconds.

Another simpler example of how we develop patterns may offer a clearer explanation: fold your arms across your chest, as you would normally do. Now stretch you hand above your head, rest them by your side and now fold your arms the opposite way. A little confusion occurs here. You may have to focus visually, as well as mentally, on what you are doing. Retraining your thinking to the new movement is unusual and requires effort. However, the next day when you fold your arms, you automatically revert to the old, set pattern. We do not want to make the extra effort. Why should we? Everything works well enough, does it not? So leave it alone!

This variation of a set pattern, however unnatural, causes confusion both physically and mentally. Its correction may take far longer than anticipated. Many people assume that when pain occurs it can be fixed immediately - permanently. A great deal of cases where pain occurs (other than sporting injuries and accidents) is the result of an accumulation of incorrect muscle control over a period of time. This gradual 'build up' of muscle imbalance can later manifest itself in one sudden occurrence as simple as turning a little further around in the car seat when you are reversing and your back 'gives way'.

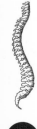

In some cases, however slight this extra, different movement is, it may be capable of causing extreme pain. The effects of chronic pain on our day to day lives can be seen in those around us. We all know someone who has pain of some kind, whether it is back pain, neck and shoulder pain or other types.

The Complete Guide to the Pilates Method

Pain can be a debilitating 'dis-ease' that can be so damaging that it can practically make a person suicidal. The relief of the pain, depending upon its severity, can be from a simple tablet to ease a headache to an operation to fuse the vertebrae in the spine.

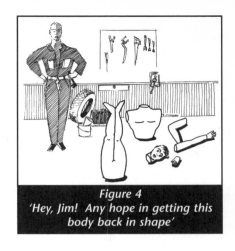

Figure 4
'Hey, Jim! Any hope in getting this body back in shape'

Loading the Body and The Stretch Factor

Prior to the aerobics craze, the introduction of the Nautilus equipment and the boom in marathon running, gyms were populated predominantly by men who wanted to show off their bulging biceps to the nearest female in sight. The females tended to gravitate towards the more feminine activities such as ballet. These activities are challenging in themselves, but did not entice the majority of the female population to donning a leotard and tights and rushing en masse into the dance studio as the aerobics phenomenon was able to do.

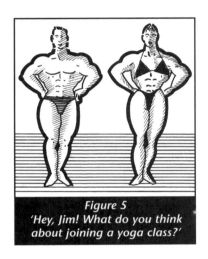

Figure 5
'Hey, Jim! What do you think about joining a yoga class?'

At almost the same time, women also discovered weight training and the effects of having stronger, more toned and well-defined bodies. Women, themselves, appreciated their latest triceps definition. The sad truth however, is that the flexibility factor was diminishing and their bodies were becoming tighter, their muscles were starting to bulge and the feminine, lithe body was beginning to disappear.

Stretching started to become more important in the return to a leaner body. Furthermore, its effectiveness in reducing injuries in sport, and physical activity in general, was earning a fast reputation. Even major league football teams began to employ ex-ballet dancers to show them how to stretch!

The effects of weight training on the gym-junkie, and certain sporting activities such as tennis or golf, create unbalanced muscle structures purely because of the nature of the action that the muscle is required to undertake. For example, the playing forearm of a world class squash player would be significantly larger than his/her non-playing arm.

In our everyday lives, not only is the body being 'loaded' by normal gravitational forces but also by unnatural forces. Forces such as movements of lifting the shopping or attending the gym, the latter sometimes imposing a greater force than the counter force required by the body to sustain a level of equilibrium - the result leading to muscle strain and possible injury. For example, lifting or bench-pressing a weight greater than that which the body is capable of sustaining. The resultant extra strain leads to torn muscles which were commanded to exert a far greater effort than they were capable of adequately supporting.

Our joints endure tremendous forces when we run, climb, jump, bend, twist, arch, push, pull and more.

These joints are practically every bone in the body that comes into contact with another bone. For example, the more common joints that we know are the elbow, shoulder, hip, knee, wrist and ankle joints. The less common joints that we tend to refer to are the joints of the fingers, toes and those of the spine (the vertebrae).

As I have mentioned above, gravity is an important 'stress' on the body. Every movement we do is against the gravitational pull of the earth. Our bodies exert a counter-action. As Isaac Newton said, "To every action, there is an equal and opposite reaction." This is true of every movement we undertake. It is at the point of a greater action, that the body can 'react' to comfortably, that the weakest joint or muscle will give way and occasionally, the strongest one cannot sustain.

The Complete Guide to the Pilates Method

Our skeletal frame is held together by muscles, tendons and ligaments. We feel overexertion as muscular strain and aching muscles. This is felt as muscle ache after a strenuous aerobics class or a long run. Too much stress or more loading than is comfortable not only stresses the muscle, but also the tendons and/or ligaments. This is felt closer to the joint and not as much in the muscle fibre. For example, the sudden loading and twisting on a skier's knee can tear the cruciate ligaments in the back of the knee and the pain is felt in the knee joint.

The direction of the forces that are placed on the joint are also a determining factor in the resultant ache or break of the muscle or bone. As in the example of the skier, he is able to reduce his chances of injury by maintaining his flexibility in his hips, knees and spine. Strength is also required in his thighs, buttocks and abdominals for a greater sense of balance when in a forward bent position. Mental alertness is an often forgotten factor in all activities. It is necessary in avoiding sudden, unexpected stresses. Mental alertness can also improve physical reflexes to avoid unusual and possibly injurious situations.

In the case of a football player, extra strength is required to protect the joints because of the extra forces placed on the body from all directions. A football player is tackled from all directions - front, back, sides and other angles and by different amounts of forces depending on the weight and size and speed of the person performing the tackle.

The Importance of Levers

If a football player were to ski and a skier were to play football, we can clearly see that further physical conditioning, strengthening and a change of mental attitude is required for each of these to perform the other's sport. The muscular and joint stresses are different and each athlete would ache after an initial training session of the other's sport. In order to understand the concept of stresses and loads on muscle groups we need to understand the principle of levers and how they relate to our bodies. In exercising, levers will help us to understand how to reduce straining certain muscles by physically (and mentally) applying effort from a stronger muscle in order to protect weaker muscles and joints from strain and injury.

Loads or weights can create additional stresses on a joint. The heavier the weight or load, the greater the muscle and surrounding structures are required to work in order to cope with the additional force (Fig. A-ii). When the muscle exerts a greater effort than the additional applied force, the body can usually cope quite comfortably and bring it to equilibrium. As the externally applied force increases, so too, does the effort required by the muscle; but only to a point. Although the externally applied force may not exceed that force exerted by the muscle, the muscle may still strain. This is dependent on the condition of the muscle and the amount of time the external force is applied. The greater the duration, the more likely the muscle will strain (Fig. B).

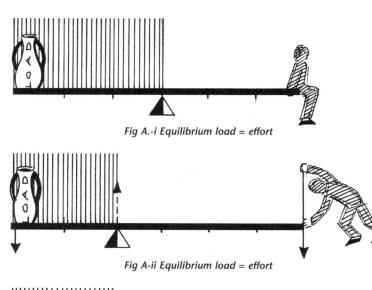

Fig A.-i Equilibrium load = effort

Fig A-ii Equilibrium load = effort

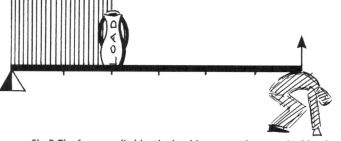

Fig B The force applied by the load is greater than required by the effort

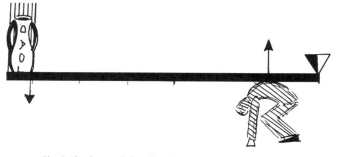

Fig C The force of the effort has to be greater than the force of the load

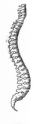

As the load applied exceeds that point at which the counter force of the muscle is able contain the weight, the effort required by the muscle has to be greater than that of the load or it may tear or rupture. This may happen immediately with an extremely heavy load and where the muscle is not warmed up such as lifting a very heavy box, the back muscles become 'overloaded' and pull (Fig. C). Or it may happen where the same weight is constantly applied over a lengthy period of time and the endurance of the muscle is no longer able to contain the stress of the weight, for example, holding a heavy wooden pole at arms length for a period of time.

Case Study

A middle-aged female attending a normal gym approached an instructor and mentioned that she had a 'weak back'. Without questioning the client as to the history of her condition, or the amount of exercise or warm-up prior to her consultation with him, the instructor placed the client on a weighted, back extension machine and asked her to complete 3 sets of 10 repetitions. This was in order to 'strengthen' her back. Before completion of her first set, she complained of more severe lower back pain. With the added resistance of the weights on the upper part of the back, the effort required to extend the back became greater than the lower back muscles could sustain and more pain was incurred. However, if the abdominal muscles were strong enough to support these lower back muscles, the effort required by the back muscles would be lessened.

In many cases of 'weak' lower backs (usually a description of pain in the area), the opposite is the case. The lower back muscles are too 'tight' and the abdominal muscles are too weak. In the above case, the client should initially have been referred to a practitioner for evaluation before commencing any loaded back exercises.

We can now see how easy it is to strain our bodies by placing forces, whether internally (by performing uncommon movements that our bodies are not capable of achieving) or externally (by outside forces such as lifting a heavy box when our body is incapable of doing so).

Our bodies require continual conditioning in order to contain the physical demands of everyday living. If we are able to mentally condition ourselves to perform basic physical conditioning routines that involve warming up, flexibility, strength and cooling down as part of a regular program, we will become increasingly mentally capable of enduring the stresses of today's living. A beneficial circle of achievement!

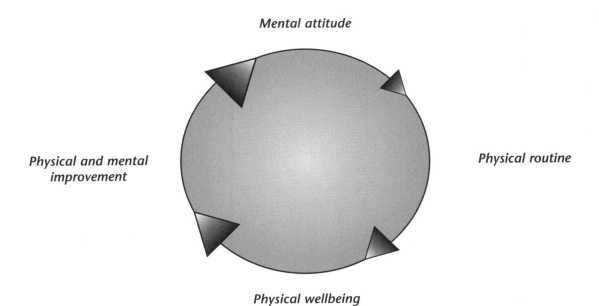

Mental attitude

Physical and mental improvement

Physical routine

Physical wellbeing

On the other hand, if our bodies are under stress, we tend to feel pain and this too can create a circle of discomfort. When we feel pain, our body's automatic reaction is to protect the injured area. For example, an injury to the shoulder. In doing so, we restrict the movement of the area for fear of doing more damage. This lack of normal mobility restricts the healing process after the acute stages of the injury. The muscle can shorten and when a normal movement from the shoulder is attempted, without adequate conditioning and rehabilitation, pain is still felt with the result being more protection of the area.

The Complete Guide to the Pilates Method

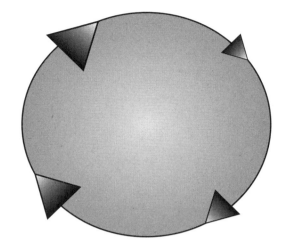

Pain or injury

Attempt at normal movement

Stiffness of the muscle or joint, lessening of blood flow

Protection (mental) = decrease in movement

To overcome this detrimental cycle, our understanding of how our bodies work and react to various stresses is important. The strengthening and stretching of our bodies, in the correct manner, is vital to break this cycle and certainly assists in the prevention of further injury to the same area, as well as other parts of our body.

As we become more aware of our bodies and how they function, we are more likely to discover hidden quirks and peculiarities. For instance, a client once said that they never realised they had back pain until it went away!

We live with many 'hidden' stresses every day. Our bodies have learned to cope with them. However, our lives would be more fulfilled if we could control many of the subconscious movements we take for granted. Movements that cause twinges (an often ignored warning of things to come?) or restrictions that prevent us doing what we once enjoyed, either sports or simply feeling more agile and alert as we grow older.

To achieve this level of wellbeing, we should be aware that it is a challenge. There are no short cuts to a better body, a new you or a sense of achieving renewed vigour and vitality at whatever age we choose. We wonder why our bodies 'fall apart' as we grow older. If we did not brush our teeth every day with a good toothbrush and paste, our teeth would eventually decay, rot and fall out. If we do not exercise our bodies regularly in the correct manner with the right techniques, our bodies too would also decay and 'fall apart'.

You can!

Well, imagine an exercise routine that can give you a firmer, flatter stomach, improve your posture, provide you with more energy and may even make you taller! Imagine an exercise routine that does not involve mindless jumping around to loud, thumping music in order to achieve the benefits of great muscle tone. Imagine an exercise routine that provides you with the stretching benefits of a yoga class and the strengthening of a gym routine. Imagine an exercise routine that provides you with the control, balance and strength of a gymnast or a competitive athlete without a steamy, 'sweat' session.

Figure 6
Lack of exercise = weak muscles

Now imagine combining all of the above into ONE exercise routine.
This is the routine that will change your life and your mental attitude to your
own body. This is a routine that can give you increased vitality, make you feel years younger and improve your posture while toning those 'flabby' muscles. This is a routine than can eliminate that nagging back pain and help you enjoy a better sex life!

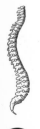

20

The Pilates Method described here is based on eight extremely sound principles. Having looked at various forms of yoga, ballet, martial arts, animal movements and strengthening programs, Josef Pilates devised his unique conditioning program. This program was simple in its theory and effective in its execution. The Pilates Method has followed traditional standard approaches devised over seventy years ago. Though brilliant in their application, some traditionalists of the Pilates Method have been reluctant to vary the original teachings.

Today we live a very different lifestyle to that of 70 years ago. Coupled with the current knowledge of the human anatomy and the body's ways of moving, the Pilates Method has formed an excellent basis for the exercises in the pages of this book.

As the Pilates Method has grown it has also evolved and with that evolution has arrived a more exact, precise and 'athletic' approach to the method. The 'balletic' approach to Pilates over the last 70 years has held the method in good stead with dancers, ex-dancers and the like. In today's environment and lifestyle, an approach requiring more knowledge in different movements required by a variety of body types is important. Hence we have not used 'models' for the poses in this book.

The exercises described in this book have been refined and enhanced over a period of fifteen years, taking into account the 'athlete' in every person. This is not to mean that the program is for athletes alone. It has been carefully designed, in various levels, for those ranging from 'basic' to 'advanced', from injured to supremely fit of any age and of any ability. It is for the 'athlete' in all of us.

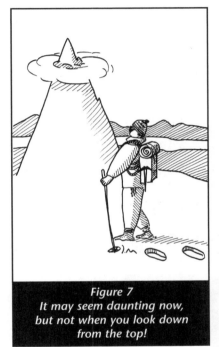

Figure 7
It may seem daunting now, but not when you look down from the top!

The Pilates Method is a safe, no-impact exercise routine that stretches and strengthens all the major muscle groups in a logical sequence, without neglecting the smaller, weaker muscles. It can be a customised program catering for the individual requirements of any body.

I have attempted to provide the most comprehensive guide to the exercises in the following pages, so that many others may experience the benefits of the Pilates Method. However, I do feel that this is no substitute for a qualified, experienced Pilates instructor or a studio registered with the Pilates Institute of Australasia.

As you will discover, the exercises are a challenge at the beginning, both physically and mentally.

Fantastic results can be achieved.

Persistence is the key.

If you think you can...

YOU CAN!

NOTES

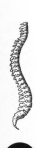

CHAPTER 2

"The science of Contrology® disproves that prevalent and all-too-trite saying 'you're only as old as you feel' " - J.Pilates

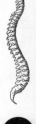

CHAPTER 2

MIND OVER MATTER - POSITIVE MENTAL ATTITUDE TO EXERCISE

We would all like a magic formula to avoid the occurrence or recurrence of any debilitating condition. The best formula for the reduction and avoidance of muscle pain is simple - exercise, mobilise, visualise. Exercising an injured part of the body, or a specific muscle, should always be achieved under the supervision of a qualified exercise oriented practitioner or qualified Pilates instructor. Keeping the joints supple without putting stress into the musculo-skeletal structure is as good, and as simple a tonic, as any. The secret lies, not in the achievement of flexibility at any cost, but in the physical control and mental understanding of the movement being performed. It has often been stated that if exercise came in a pill, it would be the most prescribed drug in the western world.

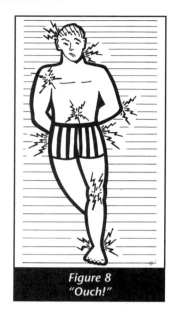

Figure 8
"Ouch!"

Before allowing our bodies to get to this 'late' stage, we are sent the occasional warning signals - the odd muscle cramp here, the unusual twinge or minor ache there. As educated adults we tend to ignore these minor signs as, 'Oh! It's nothing. It will take care of itself.' If only it would. We assume that by sitting down all day for years and then doing a quick jog around the block (without any signs of an impending heart attack) we are as fit as a fiddle and can play a three hour game of competitive tennis the next day. (The 'jog' was our self-assessment fitness test - and we passed!) Our mental power, in its limited capacity, has told us that, without any serious after effects, we have the athletic capability of a teenager.

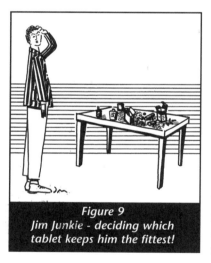

Figure 9
Jim Junkie - deciding which
tablet keeps him the fittest!

With minimal warming up and less than adequate stretching, we then proceed to push our bodies to the limits of the physical challenges of the day. We would be surprised if we were not aching the following day. 'This must be good,' we say to ourselves, 'We have worked our muscles really well.' And then, we remain inactive until the same time the following week.

The infrequency with which we tend to our bodies is scandalous. We tend to our cars better than we care for our far more complex 'machines' with so many thousands more delicate parts.

Anything more serious than the occasional ache or pain and we shuffle off to the doctor, or practitioner, who prescribes a concoction of tablets whose names we cannot pronounce, or treats the affected area, which has been aching for days, in under an hour. We feel better and assume the problem is fixed for good - we hope.

Unfortunately, for most of us, this is the start of the body telling us of the commencement of the decay process. This 'decay' does not necessarily take place throughout the entire body at the same time. It could be a knee problem here, a neck problem there. This 'decay' coincidentally occurs when we seem to slow down and not undertake regular, physical activity as we had done some years before.

Little wonder that we were able to conduct high-impact aerobic sessions with such ease and some years after we have stopped, without much strenuous activity, we are suddenly starting to fall apart.

The answer is simple. The wear and tear that the body and its joints have been subject to for many years is beginning to show through. Combine these ingredients with the lack of safe, regular stretching and conditioning programs and we have a recipe for immobility, discomfort and, too frequently, pain.

In years gone by, we were capable of pushing our bodies without too much warming up. And our bodies were able to withstand these pressures. The 'young' muscles can easily cope with spontaneous strenuous activity. The energy levels of our adolescent years seem to remain in our memory banks years after they have actually diminished.

Unfortunately, we still think we have this endless source of youthful vigour without having to work to maintain it or 'keep those batteries charged'. On a pleasant, sunny afternoon with friends we feel capable of over-reaching for that elusive kick or hit of the soccer ball, tennis ball or volleyball. Ouch! Too late. The damage is done. We feel a sharp pain in the back, hamstring or shoulder and continue to play because we are 'fit' (or so we wish to appear to those around us). The pain is bearable. We retire to bed and trust that a good night's rest will see us well in the morning. Morning arrives and - we cannot move!

These 'signs of aging' do not only affect us mere mortals. We see it in all professions. Even ballet dancers, who would be the epitome of flexibility and fitness to most of us, acquire creaky hip, knee and ankle joints later in life. No one is able to escape the advance of old age. However, there are solutions to cope with this onset of physical senility so that we are able to enjoy life in a more pain free and fulfilling manner.

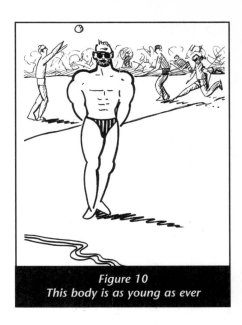

Figure 10
This body is as young as ever

THE MENTAL FACTOR

"By reawakening 1000's and 1000's of otherwise ordinary dormant muscle cells, Contrology®
correspondingly reawakens 1000's and 1000's of dormant brain cells, thus activating new areas
and stimulating further the functioning of the mind." - J.Pilates

Our general mental attitude to our bodies is one of invincibility. However, when our bodies fail us we are somewhat surprised. An injury which 'lays us low', or even hospitalises us, can be emotionally devastating. In many instances the grieving we go through after an injury has immobilised us, if we are physically active, has been paralleled to that of losing a loved one.

During the physical rehabilitation process, we generally pay considerable attention to the precise details of what is required to get us back on track. Some of us become so involved in the procedure and outcome that we become obsessed with how it all works. We become more knowledgeable about muscles, injury and the curing of our particular complaint. We become so expert in the field that we even go as far as to advise others with similar conditions!

We are more capable of achieving results after injury because we are determined to overcome this 'affliction'. We become mentally focused on our goal. This mental focus and determination can also be used when we are not injured. It can be used to prevent injuries from happening. It can help in the speedier rehabilitation after an injury. It can be used to gain greater control over weak muscle groups. It can be used to improve our performance in whatever sport or movement we desire.

Concentrating on the precision of what we are physically doing will also make us mentally alert. This takes practice and repetition. To be in control of our bodies involves understanding what we are currently capable of achieving, and how we can safely extend these limits. We need to achieve a 'thinking body' that is eventually able to control movements, however demanding, with precision, control and fluidity without having to think about what the demands of the movement are. This requires mental focus.

DEVELOPING A 'THINKING BODY'

"Contrology® begins with mind control over muscles." - J.Pilates

To develop the thinking body we need to understand the body itself; the major muscle groups and their function and how these determine physical outcome. The purpose here is to provide a broad understanding of these areas without becoming too clinical in the approach. Many of you who have suffered injuries would be familiar with these terms.

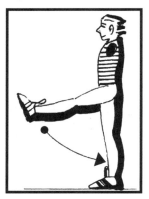

EXTENSION means lengthening out or straightening.

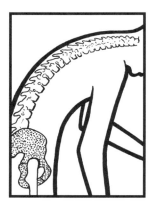

FLEXION means folding or bending. Flexors of the toes curl the toes.

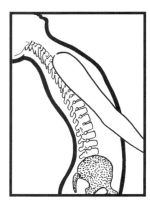

HYPEREXTENSION means extending further than 180 degrees.

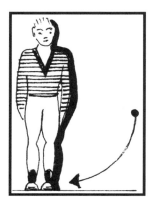

ADDUCTION means movement that draws inwards (toward the midline of the body)

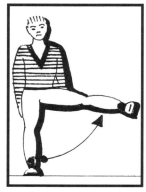

ABDUCTION means movement that draws away (from the midline of the body)

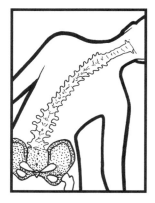

LATERAL FLEXION is a side bend of the body. Adductors and abductors oppose one another

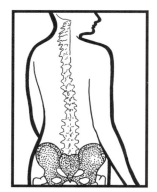

ROTATION means movement around the central axis of a lever

OTHER ANATOMICAL TERMS

Tendon: elastic connective tissue that connects muscle to bone
Ligament: non-elastic connective tissue that connects bone to bone
Lordosis: the hyperextension of the normal curve in the lumbar or cervical spine
Kyphosis: the forward flexion of the normal thoracic curve of the spine
Scoliosis: lateral curvature of the spine
Supine: on the back
Prone: on the stomach

Range of motion/movement (ROM): the degree in which a limb may comfortably move around a joint without affecting other parts of the body.

THE SKELETON

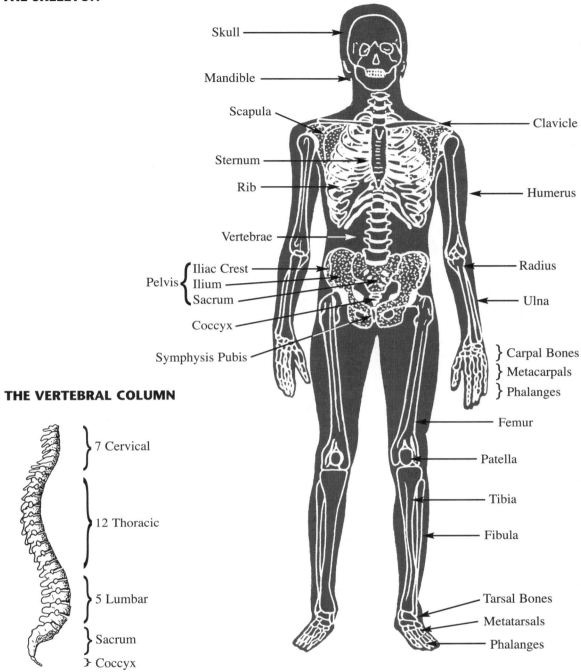

Skull
Mandible
Scapula
Clavicle
Sternum
Rib
Humerus
Vertebrae
Iliac Crest
Ilium
Pelvis
Sacrum
Radius
Coccyx
Ulna
Symphysis Pubis
Carpal Bones
Metacarpals
Phalanges
Femur
Patella
Tibia
Fibula
Tarsal Bones
Metatarsals
Phalanges

THE VERTEBRAL COLUMN

7 Cervical

12 Thoracic

5 Lumbar

Sacrum

Coccyx

The skeletal system comprises 226 bones. The important areas of mobilisation, in combination with the muscles, are all the major joints.

These joints are separated into 2 major areas
1. hinge joints : knee, elbow
2. rotational joints (ball and socket): ankle, hip, shoulder, wrist
   The entire skeleton is held together by muscles, tendons and ligaments and connective tissue. Without this the skeleton would simply fall to the floor because of the gravitational pull of the earth.

The skeleton has several important functions:
1. to act as a framework to support the softer parts of the body
2. it protects the more delicate areas of our body, such as the brain, heart, lungs and spinal cord
3. helps to produce blood cells in the bones, which contain red marrow
4. by combining with the contraction of the muscles, it allows us to move.

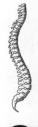

27

MAJOR MUSCLES -FRONT

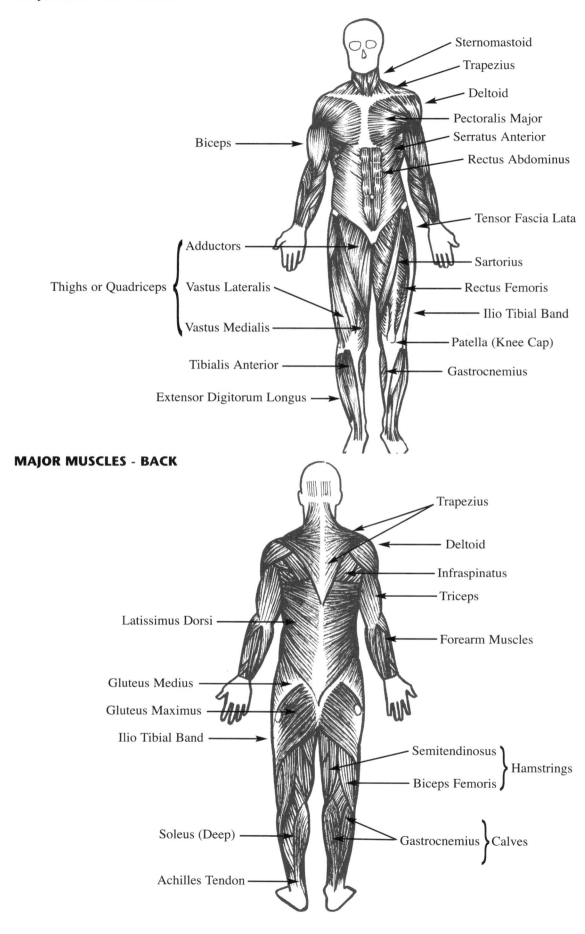

Sternomastoid

Trapezius

Deltoid

Pectoralis Major

Serratus Anterior

Rectus Abdominus

Biceps

Tensor Fascia Lata

Adductors

Sartorius

Thighs or Quadriceps {

Vastus Lateralis

Rectus Femoris

Ilio Tibial Band

Vastus Medialis

Patella (Knee Cap)

Tibialis Anterior

Gastrocnemius

Extensor Digitorum Longus

MAJOR MUSCLES - BACK

Trapezius

Deltoid

Infraspinatus

Triceps

Latissimus Dorsi

Forearm Muscles

Gluteus Medius

Gluteus Maximus

Ilio Tibial Band

Semitendinosus } Hamstrings

Biceps Femoris

Soleus (Deep)

Gastrocnemius } Calves

Achilles Tendon

The Complete Guide to the Pilates Method

THE EIGHT PRINCIPLES OF THE PILATES METHOD

To understand the Pilates Method, we first need to understand the principles behind the technique and why they are so essential. Without understanding the essentials, it is akin to attempting to drive a car without the engine; you may cruise along the flats but it becomes extremely hard work when it comes to the hills!

The manner in which the exercises are performed is of far greater importance than the number of repetitions or exertion applied to the movements. Quality is superior to quantity. Together with application and dedication to the basic principles, results can be more easily achieved. Attaining the body that one desires is not as 'scientific' or mind-bending as many people perceive.

To master a simple movement is sometimes more difficult to achieve than to force the body to perform tasks beyond its normal capabilities.

The EIGHT principles are:

> *CONCENTRATION*
>
> *BREATHING*
>
> *CENTERING*
>
> *CONTROL (inc. STRENGTH)*
>
> *PRECISION*
>
> *FLOWING MOVEMENT*
>
> *ISOLATION (inc. FLEXIBILITY)*
>
> *ROUTINE*

The above eight principles may, at first, appear simple and logical in their individual parts. It is more challenging to remember all of them at the same time when performing a simple exercise. To focus on even two of them, when beginning the program, may require some effort. Slowly, as you are able to master one principle at a time with some of the more basic exercises, you will discover the enormous impact that even a slight variation of the movement can have on the effort required to perform that movement.

> *It is the mind's subconscious control over habitual movements which needs to be altered*
> *to progress above and beyond our standard capabilities.*

As the exercises are more readily mastered, we are capable of achieving more than we have previously accomplished. This may take some time. As we follow the exercises that we find are easily performed, more challenging versions are suggested. As we perform the routines on a regular basis, we discover that at the end of a session our energy levels have increase as we achieve more. The days do not seem as long and we look forward to physical and mental challenges without regarding them as insurmountable problems. We perceive them as challenges with a natural solution. We awake more refreshed, we sleep better, our physical and mental reflexes are more highly tuned.

Frederich von Schiller, an eighteenth century German philosopher once said, 'It is the mind itself which builds the body'. With the Pilates Method, not only are we exercising our bodies, we are simultaneously exercising our minds.

1. CONCENTRATION

"Concentrate on the correct movements each time you exercise, lest you do them improperly and thus lose all the vital benefits of their value." - J.Pilates

Concentration with regard to body movement is required at all times. To focus on muscles as they move is not an easy task to master, initially, as the body does not easily follow what the mind wants it to do. If these muscles have not been often used before, the initial movement is awkward and jerky. Once continual mental attention and focus is achieved, what once appeared as simple movements actually become quite complex. The first step of the process is the realisation that the position and the movement of every part of the body is of great importance and interconnected. When walking or running, or reaching for a cup of coffee, the positioning of the foot or arm, are both influenced, and affected by, the correct alignment of the body's posture.

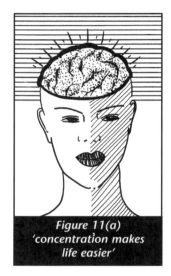

To concentrate on the entire body at the same time as it performs complex movements is a formidable challenge and takes time. It is a skill that is acquired as the method becomes more familiar. By focusing your attention on specific muscles, the mental process becomes more tuned-in. As these movements begin to achieve a level of precision the results are more noticeable. Concentration is required in the following seven principles for each movement. Each principle becomes clearer and more focused with the improved concentration that is required. Your thinking becomes clearer and you become more focused on other issues when outside the studio or exercise environment.

The benefits of concentration are somewhat obvious: clarity of thought; better mental focus leading to increased mental energy; increased ability to handle difficult situations more calmly and positively; 'fresh' approaches to new and unusual conditions, the list goes on.... You will discover, even at the start of the routines, that in order to accomplish even the most simple of exercises our minds need to focus on small movements.

Figure 11(a)
'concentration makes life easier'

Physical (restrictive) patterns that have become 'embodied' in our subconscious are in need of alteration. In some cases this can be quite demanding, requiring effort and determination to correct imbalances that have been present for months and, even, years. This focus while the body is in motion requires just that much more mental energy. Over time, like the benefits of the exercises themselves, this meditative effect slowly 'seeps' its way into the subconscious and the entire body and mind become more energised after the exercise routine.

As we correctly perform the movements we find that we are unable to think of other things that have happened during the day. We eliminate problems from our mind. We truly give this time to ourselves.

2. CENTERING

The abdominal area is often described as the second spine. It is the powerhouse of the anatomy. The centre is described as the area between the ribs and the hips at both anterior (front) and posterior (back) parts of the torso. A strong centre is also important to maintaining good control and balance in the body as a whole. It provides assistance for movements both slow and fast, such as balancing on a beach ball or sprinting the 100 meters.

Imagine a ballet dancer standing on one leg on pointe (of the foot), with the other leg in the air to the ceiling and her arms above the head - and loose abdominals (or worse still, a potbelly!). She would fall over instantly. The centre is the pivotal point of the body.

Figure 11(b)
"Dancer - pot belly"

All strength movements emanate from this area. In karate, the Ki comes from the solar plexus. The effort of movement, force, balances and strength comes from the centre.

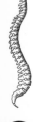

Abdominal control is different to abdominal strength. However, the former does rely on the latter. It is preferable to have the former. In many workout routines, most of the abdominal strength is achieved by performing 'crunches', sit-ups or some manner of forward 'contraction' or flexion of the body. This limits the control of the abdominals and most of it's strength to that position where the abdominal contraction takes place. ie. a forward curved position of the torso; abdominal strength provides support, abdominal control provides fluidity of movement from the centre.

Case Study

Tennis players do most of their abdominal strength work by performing crunches with knees bent. When they stand up the abdominal muscles are more lengthened and have less strength than the position in which they were worked. As a result, when performing their serve, the abdominal muscles are at full stretch. There is no strength from their centre to perform this movement efficiently and effectively. The majority of the force for the serve then comes from the shoulder and arm. If the abdominals were strengthened when at full stretch, the centre can be brought into play and the serve become more effective. The same applies to the majority of sports.

THE 'B-LINE'

This is an age old Pilates approach to abdominal control, however there is more emphasis placed here on the exactness of the movement and how best to engage the lower abdominals. The B-Line, together with correct foot placement, is the foundation of good posture. (See Chapter 3 - Tripods)

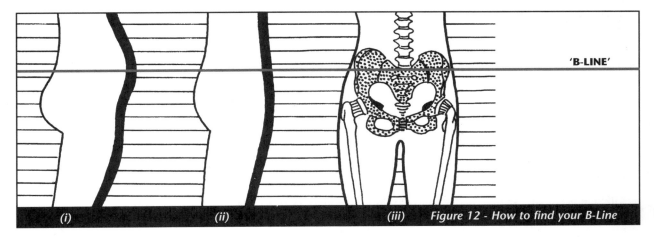

'B-LINE'

(i)   (ii)   (iii)   *Figure 12 - How to find your B-Line*

1. Stand upright with feet hip distance apart
2. Draw the abdominals as close to the spine as possible and breathe normally

What do you feel?

You may notice several things occur here:

1. the area drawing to the spine is generally the navel, or mid and upper abdominals with some lower abdominal connection
2. the pelvis may be tucked to provide a feeling of 'flattening' the back (this especially happens when lying on the floor or standing against a wall
3. the knees may bend slightly or the shoulders round. The ribs slightly drop to the hips
4. the buttock may be clenched
5. the breathing may be somewhat restricted with a feeling of forcing the breath into the lungs
6. there is generally little or no feeling of abdominal contraction in the area below the navel

Now abolish all thoughts of navel to spine!

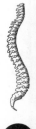

Stand as before and relax. Now:

1. With your finger, trace a straight line from the top of one hipbone to the other (see diagram). You may notice that line is in front of the hipbones (Fig.13(i)).
2. Go to the centre of this line (5 to 8 centimetres below the belly button) and draw the stomach in BEHIND the LINE of the hips (hence, B-Line) and away from your finger.

> **Without -**   **i)**   clenching the buttocks
>   **ii)**   tucking the pelvis or
>   **iii)**   dropping the shoulders.

When was the last time you felt *these* lower abdominal muscles working!

This is the B-Line - "MAINTAIN THIS FOR THE REST OF YOUR LIFE!!"
We shall be using this term throughout the book.
Initially, there may be some mild discomfort in the lower back. This will diminish as the body is used to this new positioning. You may notice that you may be standing a little more upright! The breathing may still be restricted - Breathe as described in the following section.

AN EXAMPLE OF THE B-LINE IN ACTION:

Stand up out of a chair. You may notice that the upper body may have leant forward over the knees first, before coming to the standing position. Take a seat again and now B-Line before you rise up out of the chair. You may notice that you stood up without leaning forward so far, and your back may have felt more supported.

THE PERFECT ABDOMINAL CURL - PAC

When working the abdominal muscles to gain strength in exercises involving a forward contraction, such as roll-ups, sit-ups or maintaining a contracted position, there is a definite sequence of movements to follow.

The first movement, even before the head is raised off the floor, is 'B-Line'. This also has a significant benefit in that it creates pressure against the psoas (see 'Muscle Imbalances' p.44) and reduces its pull, thereby reducing stiffness, or an arch, in the lower back. The tailbone is not tilted to the ceiling. This gives a false impression of keeping the back flat.

1. Keep the knees bent at a right angle at the knee joint, or further, as long as the lower back remains flat, without tucking the pelvis or pressing the feet into the floor. Keep the feet flexed and the eyes above the knees.

2. Draw the rib cage towards the hips and scoop the abdominals. This action then brings the head and shoulders forward without the usual strain in the neck. When performing the curl the ribs are drawn towards the hips as close as possible in a horizontal plane, taking a deep sigh out. The return is a release of only 10% of the contraction before repeating the movement. The shoulder blades should never rest on the floor at any time until all repetitions are complete. If they do, they 'release' the control of the abdominals and they almost rest!

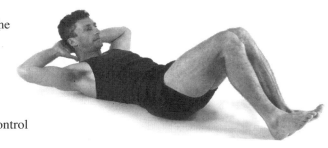

Nine times out of ten, the usual crunch is performed by first lifting the head and shoulders forward to perform the movement. By allowing this reflex action to dominate, the abdominals usually bulge out, and after a while, the neck and shoulders start to strain. In many cases, people have said that they perform hundreds of crunches but still have back pain! As long as the ribs are drawn to the hips in the same plane, with the abdominals scooped (try to imagine copying a greyhound's stomach!), the abdominals will perform their function correctly. When the ribs lift above the level of the hips, then the hip flexors engage and the back stiffens to perform a lift. The purpose of the curl is then defeated, and the abdominals do not perform to 100% capacity.

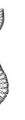

3. BREATHING

"To breathe correctly you must completely exhale and inhale, always trying very hard to 'squeeze' every atom of impure air from your lungs in much the same manner that you would wring every drop of water from a wet cloth." - J.Pilates

Breathing is the most important physical principle to refine before attempting an exercise or movement. It is vital to learn to breathe correctly.

Breathing has three major functions:
1. to carry nutrients to all parts of the body thereby 'charging' the body's whole with more energy
2. to carry away wastes for elimination from the body
3. to increase stamina.

The wastes can produce 'restrictions' within the body's system. These can be various, such as tightness and restricted movement in joints, tiredness, headaches and pain. This is not to say that breathing on its own can cure these 'ailments'. It cannot. Combined with the other principles it can certainly lead to greater wellbeing. Drinking the required quantity of water (eight glasses per day), to assist in the waste elimination process also assists greatly towards this goal. It has also been suggested that adequate water consumption can improve flexibility of the muscles.

As we have all seen in gym and other (weight) training situations, many fitness attendees hold their breath at the most crucial part of the exercise when it can be most beneficial. We have probably been guilty of this ourselves, in the past, without realising it. By doing this we put our bodies under an enormous amount of physical tension, especially in the upper thoracic and cervical area.

Holding the breath while exercising is similar to pressure building up inside a pressure cooker. As a result, energy and effort are wasted on a part, or parts, of the body where they are not required. The outcome is less than efficient utilisation of the muscles being worked as the subconscious, mental concentration becomes more focused on the stress the body is undergoing.

Try this simple exercise. Breathe in as you raise your arms above your head. Press your arms to your sides, as if through a vat of treacle. As you lower them and hold your breath for as long as you can. Can you feel the tension in the neck and shoulders? Now repeat the same exercise, but when you have breathed in, gradually let the breath out in a long sigh. Can you feel how much more relaxing this is?

Correct breathing should be performed with the following in mind:

1. **Keep the neck and shoulders relaxed** - hunching causes neck tension
2. **Allow the breathing to flow** - don't hold the breath at any point
3. **Breathe in through the nose** (into the chest) for a five-second count, without allowing the shoulders to lift at all (try this in front of a mirror and keep an eye on your shoulders), then without stopping
4. **Breathe out of the mouth** with a sigh for a 5-second count (drop the jaw and do not purse the lips into any shape). Blowing out of the mouth, or through the teeth, does not allow all the air to be expelled from the bottom of the lungs. It also tenses the neck, jaw and face. This unnecessary 'contortion' of the breathing leads to wastage of energy in an area that is not required to be worked. This energy can be better utilised in the performance of the exercise itself.
5. If you find it difficult to breathe into the chest, **breathe 'into your back'** or shoulderblades as if there were a deflated balloon in this area. It is often forgotten that a whole section of space exists in the back of our chest cavity for extra breath intake!

Try this (with the B-Line) as in the following exercise. See how less restricted it is and a deeper breath can be taken. This is important to increase lung capacity and improve stamina.

BREATHING EXERCISE:

Sit down with your legs comfortably crossed in front of you. Sit as upright as possible, as if your lower back were being supported by a wall, with no gaps between your tailbone and the wall. Do not lean into the wall. Place your hands snugly just below your navel. Without hunching the shoulders, take a 5-second breath in through the nose and a five-second sigh out of the mouth. You may notice that on the breath in you felt the stomach move outward. On the breath out it went down. (If 5 seconds is too long for the breath in, attempt 4 seconds.)

Now repeat the same exercise, except that before you breathe in, press your hands very firmly (on the B-Line below the navel against your lower abdominals towards your spine) and keep them there. Now breathe into your chest. You will find that this is quite difficult to achieve without the hands moving at all. You may also find that the breath into the chest may have been quite restricted and that there was a slight sensation of 'choking' the breath into your chest.

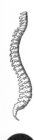

Figure 13
Restricted breathing

This is because, as we reduce our exercise levels, our breathing capacity reduces. If we return to our usual level of exercise after a long break we find that, in a short space of time, we are gasping for breath. As we tend to do less abdominal work, we tend to breathe more into the stomach and thus loosen the abdominal muscles. As this happens, our usually pliable, intercostal muscles between our ribs tighten. As they tighten they do not allow our ribs to move as much as before and, therefore, create the sensation of wearing a corset around our thoracic (chest) region when we take that deep breath into the chest. This is why there is the 'choking', restricted sensation when breathing in.

Endurance, or stamina, is the body's ability to achieve more performance over a greater length of time with less stress and fatigue. By controlling the breath at the abdominals and expanding the lung capacity, greater stamina can be achieved. It is often thought that only aerobic activity can increase stamina. However, deeper, controlled breathing, combined with even 'low grade', or non-aerobic physical activity is also capable of achieving increased stamina. As you are able to achieve a certain level of exercise with ease, increase the repetitions without resting. Performing these over a period of time, with the same initial ease, will increase muscle endurance and tone.

Case Study

Opera singers often feel uncomfortable about strengthening or tightening their stomach muscles. This is because they use the diaphragm to control their voice projection. In instances when opera singers have followed the Pilates Method, they felt that their singing had actually improved with greater abdominal control.

Over several months, as their stomach muscles improved and strengthened, the effect of 'forcing' the deeper breathing into the lungs and chest cavity also 'stretched' the intercostal muscles. With better abdominal strength, which they could now control, and increased lung capacity they were able to hold notes for longer periods as well as use the previously, barely existent abdominals for better voice projection.

Similarly, generally non-active people have reported increased stamina when going for what was once a strenuous half hour walk. After several weeks of the Pilates Method, they discovered that a ONE and a half hour walk was not particularly demanding. Their muscle tone had increased and their ability to walk a greater distance with less stress or strain also improved.

Controlled, slow, deep breathing during exercising also has the effect of becoming the norm when at rest. This is not only less stressful on the body as a whole, but those with slower (resting) breaths per minute also can have a slower resting heart rate. This can also be a determining factor in the longevity of an individual.

There are several ways to overcome the previously mentioned tightness in the chest. Here we shall explain two simple methods to assist in deeper breathing.

1. Repeat the sitting posture as above with the hands pressed firmly below the navel. Now instead of breathing into the chest, breathe 'into your back'. This concept may be difficult to attain at first. If so, try breathing into your shoulder blades (without rounding your shoulders, looking down, or collapsing your chest). This achieves the same result and more. You will find that after a few attempts, the breathing is deeper and the former, restricted breath into the chest has diminished a great deal. You may also find that, though you breathe easier, it is still not totally into the chest, but more into the sides, under the arms. This is a good start to stretching those tight intercostals. Breathe in and out ten times, to a 5 second count breath in and a 5 second count for the out breath. This shall be the standard breathing for the majority of the exercises described in this book. So, whenever there is a tight sensation on the breathing - breathe 'into your back'.

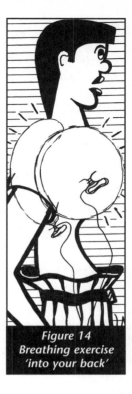

Figure 14
Breathing exercise
'into your back'

2. The second method of attaining the correct breathing control and position is to kneel on the floor on your haunches with your chest on your thighs, and your forehead rested on the floor, or on cushions for more comfort.

Place your hands as high up on your back, on the ribs, as you can without any tension in the neck or shoulder areas. In this position it would be fairly difficult to take a deep breath into the chest as it is pressed against your thighs. Now breathe into your hands. This has the same effect as breathing into the back. Try not to breathe into the chest or the abdominal area. Practice these for ten breaths in and out.

GENERAL BREATHING RULES

There are three general breathing rules to follow when performing any of the movements. (There are always some exceptions to the rules which we shall point out as they occur.)

1. When lying on the back (supine):
a. When the arms or the legs move vertically away from the centre, **breathe OUT**.
When the arms or the legs move vertically towards the centre, **breathe IN**.

AT ALL TIMES KEEP THE B-LINE.

EXERCISE:

Lie on your back on the floor with your knees bent and hands placed by your sides, palms upwards. Extend one leg into the air and slowly lower this leg away from you, breathing out. (For those with stronger abdominals, try this example with both legs in the air.) The same can be done with the arms in the air and stretching them towards the floor above the head.

As you lower the arms/legs vertically away from your centre you may notice one of two things.

i) You may actually want to breathe IN, as it may feel 'unnatural' to breathe out.
ii) As the arm/leg lowers to the floor the lower back may have a tendency to arch. B-Line when you feel this happening. You have gone as far as you are able to comfortably. Do not attempt to lower past this point. Further abdominal control is required to lower the arm/leg further without the back arching.

If you breathe IN as you lower the arms/legs, not only does the lower back have a tendency to arch, but notice that the rib cage also has a tendency to poke up into the air.

Now breathe OUT as you extend the arms/legs away and concentrate on keeping the back as flat as possible and flatten your rib cage as if a large weight has been placed on it. As the same time, to keep the back flat, press your abdominal muscles to the floor and feel them tighten. Imagine your arms/legs floating towards the floor. Can you feel how this has a greater stabilising effect on the spine? Can you feel how the abdominals and ribs work harder to maintain this position? Can you feel how your back is more supported without much stress on the spine?

1b. When the arm or legs move laterally (out to the sides) away from the midline of the body, **breathe in**.

For example when performing 'flies' with the arms to the ceiling; Breathe in as the arms open out to the sides and breathe out as they come back to the centre

2. When lying in the side position or on stomach position (prone):

Whatever is lifted against gravity, **B-Line** and **breathe OUT**. Breathe in when lowering to the floor.

3. When on all fours (hands and feet/knees):

For most movements drawing away from the centre or elongating the body, breathe IN. When closing towards the centre, keep the navel firmly to the spine and Breathe OUT. For example, see leg pull front. Exercise # 54.

4. CONTROL

"Ideally, our muscles should obey our will. Reasonably, our will should not be dominated by the reflex actions of our muscles." - J.Pilates.

Once the previous principles gave been practised and mastered as best as possible, the next principle of CONTROL can be more easily applied and utilised. Maintaining control for every movement takes concentration, effort and awareness of what the rest of the body is doing at the same time.

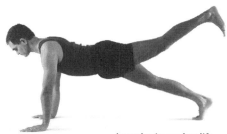
breathe in on leg lift

Whether the movements are simply lengthening the neck to reduce cervical lordosis (and maintaining that position) or a larger movement, such as a grande ronde de jamb in classical dance, the degree of control required may be the same. When these movements were initially started they took effort and concentration to perfect them to the best of the person's ability. Repetition, dedication and application improve the degree of control and the perfection of the movement.

Uncontrolled, 'automatic' movements, such as rapid lat pull-downs with weights equipment or some aerobics classes, can lead to injury as incorrect muscles are employed and incorrect posture is enforced. The action becomes mindless. Without concentration and control the body's stronger muscles will tend to do all the work (and stay stronger) and the weaker, usually 'flabby' muscles tend to remain relatively unused and remain weak.

Thus, it is control over weaker parts of the body which improves their strength. Strength can also be improved in the major muscle groups (which may already have a certain degree of strength), by increasing the load on the muscle and attempting to maintain the control over the movement as when the load was lighter. This is usually achieved by increasing the load by small amounts. The greater the load, the less the control.

When muscles are in continual motion they are being toned. When there is no control (no toning 'connection'), they are under-utilised. So, in broad terms,

If you are not toning a muscle, you are flabbing it.

If there is difficulty mentally 'feeling' the weak muscles, then follow this suggestion. Place your fingers into the weak/soft/flabby muscle to create a mental connection. (E.G. Fig.15 the inner thigh, when performing single leg circle Exercise # 22). Press the fingers against the muscle when taking the leg out to the side and press the muscle against the fingers when drawing the leg to the centre. This will give a better connection to the muscle you really want to work, rather than overworking the quadriceps muscle.

Figure 15
Fingers in muscle

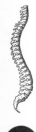

36

Control is essential to reduce and prevent injuries. Control does not necessarily mean a reduction in performance. As the initial movements are slower to gain control, some performance may be compromised. When these movements are perfected, more speed can be introduced and the previous levels of performance are superseded.

Case study

A sprinter, who attended the Body Control Pilates Studios, used to come out of the starting blocks with a 'stammering' start - very small steps until she got into her proper stride. She felt she was losing that fraction of a second as a result - and, therefore, not winning as many races! When initial work was performed to correct this imbalance in the pelvic area, her times decreased. With more specific pelvic stabilisation work, better control and strength in the pelvic area was achieved. Her times also improved! She no longer stammered out of the blocks!

---

5. PRECISION

"Correctly executed and mastered to the point of subconcsious reaction, these exercises will reflect grace and balance in your routine activities." - J.Pilates

Precision of movement leads to more graceful movements. We see this with classic ballet dancers who are required to fine tune their bodies in order to achieve an exactness of a simple, or even complex series, of jumps, port de bras or plies, or in gymnasts who require perfect balance and control when performing on the balance beam or parallel bars. When performing all these movements in a group, as in synchronised swimming, we can see the beauty, grace, style and apparent effortlessness that is the result of the precise actions of the participants.

Precision requires thought (back to that essential principle of concentration) and mental feedback (visualising and understanding what the perfect movement is). Our bodies require this feedback to let us know that we are achieving results. It is usually very difficult to obtain this feedback when working weaker muscle groups, as the stronger ones prefer to do most of the workload.

Precision of movement can also be accomplished in short actions, such as a weight trainer lifting a heavy weight or a body builder performing on stage. Precision requires controlled action without which the movement becomes sloppy and aesthetically unappealing. The space within which you move and perform various physical activities also determines, and is determined by precision.

This is very obviously seen in a gymnastic performance on a balance beam and the same gymnast performing a floor routine. One performance is a very confined and restricted (closed physical movement), the other very open and generally unrestricted (open physical movement). Both, however, require precision to achieve the goals required. Precision also requires correct positioning prior to commencing the movement to attain better performance.

6. FLOWING MOVEMENT

"Contrology® is designed to give you suppleness, natural grace and skill that will be unmistakebly reflected in (all you do)." - J.Pilates

Fluidity of movement while exercising leads to fluidity of movement when not exercising. Conscious muscular control through all ranges of movement will help eliminate stiff, jerky movements. It is in the extreme ranges of movement (ROM) that less control is likely to occur, as muscles tend to be weaker in elongated positions. Less flowing movement occurs as a result.

For example, when extending the leg or arm to kick or punch, the fast movement at the extremity (end of range) can produce a 'snapping' effect in the knee or elbow joint. Continuous repetitions of this action can result in pain in the joint. This 'snapping' of the joint is also an indication that the muscles are not in as complete control as one would expect.

This sharp movement can, and should, be eliminated to reduce any long-term wearing effect on the joint. If caused by hyperextension of the joint, then extension should only occur to the point where the joint is 'unlocked' (not noticeably bent). To a person with hyperextension, the joint would feel quite bent. However, from a normal visual approach these limbs would appear straight.

Stiff movements also occur in muscles that are too tight. We often see this with body builders who lift extremely heavy weights. They walk with short, restricted movements. The biceps muscles are so tight that the arm is continuously bent and gives the appearance of a gorilla's arm posture. Therefore, fluid movement may initially require a shortening of overextended muscles and a lengthening of the tight ones.

Make the movement continuous rather than stopping even for a fraction of a second. Continue the movements as if ten repetitions were one, rather than one repetition repeated ten times.

7. ISOLATION

"...each muscle may cooperatively and loyally aid in the uniform development of all our muscles." - J.Pilates

Once there is better control of the weaker muscle group, more control over that muscle can be obtained and increased isolation of that muscle can be achieved. Enhanced precision of movement is then also possible.

Attempt this movement, for example. Lie on your back - keep your arms slightly bent at the elbow with the palm of the hand facing the floor. Now attempt to isolate and tighten the triceps muscle of your weaker arm. Do not straighten the arm, hunch the shoulder, clench the fist or make the forearm become rigid. Do not press the arm onto the floor. (For those of you with good body awareness and physical conditioning, this may not be too difficult, so attempt the same with the hamstring of the weaker leg, the lower abdominals, the weaker rhomboid or some other weaker part of the body.)

Can you feel the triceps tighten?

For many of you it may be quite difficult to engage that triceps muscle, let alone feel where it is. The first response is to use all of the above *negative* muscular reactions to feel the contraction of the triceps. Some of you may be somewhat confounded that you cannot feel anything at all!

Now, touch the triceps with gentle pressure with your other hand and tighten the triceps. The reaction this time may be instantaneous. The connection is made. The physical contact, or touch response, provides the simple biofeedback necessary to make the mental/physical connection possible. Without the touch response it was difficult to obtain a good connection of the muscle, or even identify where the muscle was located. Now, take this a step further. Press the triceps with more force as if you were pressing the bone of the humerus (upper arm) itself. Now tighten the triceps. The reaction of the muscle is even better. For those unable to obtain the connection, do not despair. It may take several attempts for the muscle to respond. This is usually a result of not working the muscle often enough.

This increase in pressure results in a better response because we are attempting to work from the core of the muscle itself. This increase in receptivity of the muscle function leads to faster results than if the muscle were not being touched at all. Generally, the stronger muscles groups will do the majority of the work in any movement. Concentration alone may not be enough to fire those receptors to engage the weaker muscles that require toning or strength. The touch response may need to be utilised for several weeks on the same muscle before even the slightest reaction occurs. A muscle does not need to hurt or be sore the next day to know that it is working. The firmness of the muscle, or the speed with which it responds, is a good indication that it works well.

Once better control is gained over the weaker muscle, the physical contact is no longer required to 'feel' the muscle working. Together with isolation is flexibility of the limb, lever or joint. If we are better able to isolate a part of the body and allow it to move 'independently' from other parts, we are in a better position to be able to introduce more flexibility to that area (assuming we have only muscular, and not structural/bony, restrictions).

Flexibility is defined as 'the range of movement of a specific joint or group of joints influenced by the associated bones and bony structures and the physiological characteristics of the muscles, tendons, ligaments, and various other collagenous tissues surrounding the joint'. (Modern Principles of Athletic Training. Arnheim)

All of the above principles combined can lead to increased flexibility of the joints. Further means of achieving flexibility, such as specific muscle stretching techniques, can also obtain greater results. Utilising the above principles can also result in better physical performance. I have devoted an entire section to flexibility and stretching as this is extremely important in the prevention of injuries (see 'The Warm-Up' p.70-80).

Too much flexibility can lead to loss of muscular control (leading to injury) and too little can restrict movement (also leading to injury). In the former, classical ballet dancers are generally thought to be extremely flexible. However, they feel they require more strength in the extreme ranges of movement without compromising their flexibility or building bulk. At the other end of the spectrum, triathletes feel they are too tight and would certainly desire more flexibility without compromising their strength and thereby achieve better times.

8. ROUTINE

"Patience and persistence are vital qualities in the ultimate successful accomplishment of any worthwhile endeavour." - J.Pilates

Establishing a regular routine, whether it is daily or three times a week, can undoubtedly achieve greater results. Many times the question is asked, 'How long will it take me to get fit?', 'How often should I exercise?' The answer is relative to the person asking the question. Would you like to become as fit as your next door neighbour who may not consider himself fit at all?

An established Pilates routine will improve mental and physical conditioning in all individuals. The more you do - the better the result. A simple analogy would be playing the piano. To most of us this would seem a daunting task. But even the world's maestros started from scratch.

Their perseverance, dedication, energy and regular practice made them what they were. The same applies to all professions. One practice session a week will achieve far less than two, three or four times a week. The more you do - the better the result. Your sense of wellbeing will be vastly improved and you will see the world through different eyes.

The workout, including stretches, should last between 1 to 1 1/4 hours. Two workout sessions per week to start are a good effort. Three workouts per week are excellent! The gradual improvement as you master the exercises, will build your mental confidence in what you are able to achieve physically. This system of muscle conditioning, of combining the focused mental concentration with the physical aspects described above, can produce a lean, defined, muscularly balanced physique. I often mention to clients not to think of this as exercise (especially when they blow their breath out through pursed lips), but to think of this simply as movement. Movement that is fluid, unforced, but precise and controlled. Don't be surprised if you do not see much result for up to two months. As mentioned earlier, the method works from the inside out. To engage muscles that you never knew even existed takes time. On the other hand you may be surprised at how soon the results will appear!

When performing the exercises imagine that they are everyday movements, not enforced exercises. Imagine the improved control these movements can then induce in normal activity such as walking up stairs and feeling the hamstrings firmly in control. Imagine picking up a baby and feeling the abdominal muscles supporting the back or even lifting an object from an awkward position and feeling in total control of all the fibres in your body! All without having to think about these connections happening!

This is what the Pilates Method is all about, improved quality of movement that can lead to greater quality of life. Your life is in your hands. Grasp it with enthusiasm and change the way you think, feel and react to all around you.

The Complete Guide to the Pilates Method

NOTES

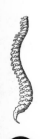

CHAPTER 3

"Controlgy® develops the body uniformly, corrects wrong postures, restores physical vitality, invigorates the mind, and elevates the spirit." - J.Pilates

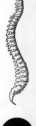

CHAPTER 3

POSTURE

Posture and physique are sometimes seen to be interdependent. It is not necessarily true to state that the better your physique, the better your posture.

BODY TYPES

According to the Sheldon classification, there are three basic human types:

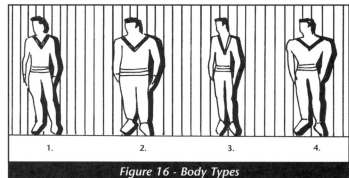

Figure 16 - Body Types

1. the **average** person would lie between the ectomorph and the mesomorph.
2. **endomorph** (larger than average - soft, large abdomen, high shoulders)
3. **ectomorph** (thin muscles and small bones, with drooped shoulders)
4. **mesomorph** (large thorax, slender waist, thick abdominal muscles)

FACTORS INFLUENCING POSTURE

Any of the above could have good or bad posture. Adult posture is more inclined to be dependent on

1. **inherited conditions**
   where genetic makeup determines the height, types of bone structure, etc. that an individual possesses
2. **habit**
   from occupational or repetitive movements, muscle function becomes restrictive, altering postural alignment
3. **disease**
   whether muscular or structural (as in bone deformity) certainly alters one's stance - limitations are then imposed on one's normal activity.

We have already discussed the effects of gravity on the muscles. They are constantly being pulled downwards. Our bodies are required to counter these forces with healthy, strong muscle structures to maintain 'good posture' and ward off the effects of strain and injury.

WHAT IS CORRECT POSTURE?

In order to discuss postural deviation, we need to understand what is meant by normal posture. When standing upright we need to imagine a plumb line through our bodies:

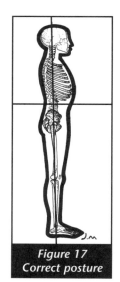

1. from side (lateral) view - from the top of our skull hanging through the centre of our body to the floor. This plumb line should pass through our centre of gravity. It passes through the ear lobe, centre of the tip of the shoulder, hip joint, behind the patella of the knee and mid-way between the heel and the balls of the foot.

2. from the back (posterior) view - the plumb line should fall through the centre of the scull, following the line of the spine, hips (between the cheeks of the buttocks) and to the floor with the lower limbs equally placed on either side of the line, with the knees and heels directly below the hips. The knees, pelvis and shoulders should also be at horizontal levels to the floor.

Figure 17
Correct posture

Our centre of gravity should lie along the intersection of these two lines and a third line that is found in the section between our hips and our lower ribs.

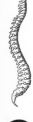

42

THE MAIN MUSCLE GROUPS WHICH CONTROL POSTURE IN A STANDING POSITION:

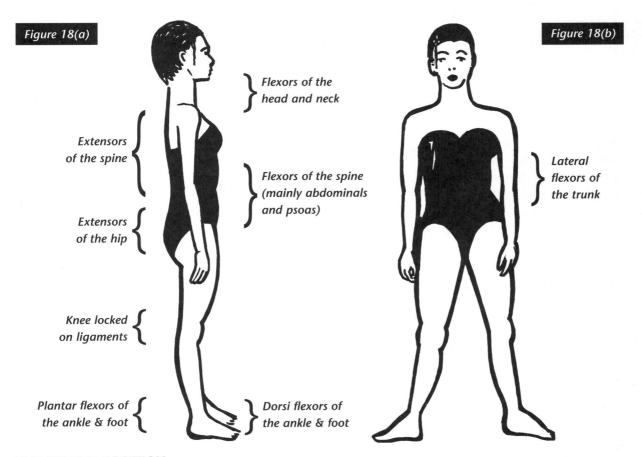

Figure 18(a)

Flexors of the head and neck

Extensors of the spine

Flexors of the spine (mainly abdominals and psoas)

Extensors of the hip

Knee locked on ligaments

Plantar flexors of the ankle & foot

Dorsi flexors of the ankle & foot

Figure 18(b)

Lateral flexors of the trunk

THE TRIPOD POSITION

The overall balance of the body (in a standing position) should be where the feet evenly support the body when they are placed directly under the hip joints. The placement of the body's weight should be evenly distributed over the three points that form a triangle on the feet: the points being - 1) the ball of the big toe, 2) the outside edge of the foot and 3) the centre of the heel. There should be no pressure forward on the toes or backward on the heels. By also placing an equal pressure on the outside edge of the foot, you may feel as if you are creating an arch where the arch should be! Try to maintain the Tripod position whenever standing.

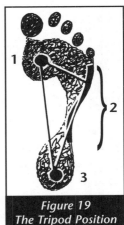

Figure 19
The Tripod Position

POSTURAL ASSESSMENT

Correct posture may be determined by either visual means or by actual measurement when the eye cannot detect slight misalignments. The two main areas where the posture can deviate from the norm are:

1. The lower limbs - feet, tibia/fibula, knee joint and femur
2. The pelvis and torso - the pelvis and the lumbar, thoracic and cervical sections of the spine and rib cage.

Bad posture in the lower limbs can emanate from conditions such as:

1. i) foot pronation or supination, inversion or eversion
   ii) knock knees (genu valgum) and bow legs (genu varum)
   iii) hyperextended or hyperflexed knees,
   iv) leg length differences
   v) tibial torsion (when the feet are parallel and the knees roll in).

The first two can be visually determined from a front view and the third from a side view.

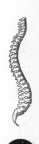

2. **i)** anterior (forward) or posterior (backward) tilt of the pelvis
   ii) lumbar lordosis
   iii) kyphosis
   iv) cervical lordosis
   v) scoliosis

3. Back view with actions of the scapula (shoulderblade) and shoulder such as:
   vi) elevation - hunched
   vii) depression - pushed down
   viii) adduction - squeezed together
   ix) abduction - winged shoulderblades
   x) forward rotation of the shoulders.

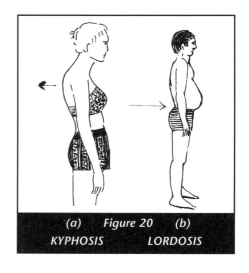

(a)   Figure 20   (b)
KYPHOSIS   LORDOSIS

Side viewing can detect positions i-iv, and x; while viewing from the back can detect v-ix).

BAD POSTURE AND ITS CONNECTION TO LOWER BACK PAIN

The following is a common example of how bad posture can affect the lower back. Simply stand with your hands on your hips. This simple, innocent movement has no less than FOUR detrimental effects on the body.

You will notice that the hands are usually placed with the fingers on the front of the hips and the thumbs 'hooked' at the top of the hip bones at the back. Most people adopt this stance, especially if they have lower back pain.

Others may adopt the 'pregnancy' stance by placing the hands in the small of the back and pushing forward, creating a large arch in the lower back.

In the long term both stances, especially the pregnancy stance, cause the following in most individuals:

The pelvis tilts forward leading to:

1. the lower back arching and these muscles become shorter and tighter
2. the thigh muscles shorten and draw the pelvis further forward, 'locking' the hips. This is commonly seen in men with beer guts who are unable to tilt the pelvis backwards
3. loosening and stretching the lower abdominals
4. hunching the shoulders leading to tighter neck muscles.

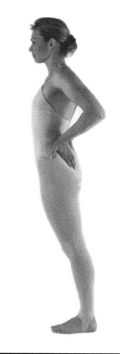

Figure 21
Pregnancy Stance

MUSCLE IMBALANCES

Muscles which overwork or strain on a frequent basis can generally cause an imbalance of the skeletal structure. It is commonly assumed that overworked muscles need stretching and under-worked muscles require strengthening for the body to be in a position of balance or equilibrium. Postural defects that can be corrected are those which are created by weak or over-strong muscles. Structural problems invariably require more than muscle reconditioning to alleviate the problem, and indeed, to correct the posture.

The hip flexors have an enormous effect on the body's structure, especially its posture. The psoas major and iliacus, if over-strong, tend to 'lift or lurch' the body from a flat (supine) position to sitting upright.

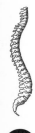

44

In order to 'roll' the spine into an upright position, these hip flexors need to be controlled by producing more mid- and lower abdominal strength.

Another group of hip flexors is the quadriceps. There are four (Latin-quad) major groups of muscles in the thigh. They attach from the top of the hip and femur to the patella and quadriceps tendon. As they are the largest group of muscle in the body, they tend to do a great deal of work without any conscious effort involved.

From when we are babies, with our legs in the air, to the time we crawl, to the time we stand erect to walk, run or jump they are continuously engaged.

If they are continually exposed to over-exertion without 'opposite relief', such as stretching, they can cause problems such as back pain.

When the muscles of the upper thigh are over-strong they tend to tilt the pelvis in an anterior position. This, in turn tends to create a small arch in the lower back, lengthening the lower abdominals and causing the iliopsoas hip flexors to also shorten and accentuate the arch in the small of the back. Although the mid and upper abdominals may appear flat, they may not be working hard enough to counter the strength of the hip flexors pulling the spine forward. This imbalance can cause considerable back pain.

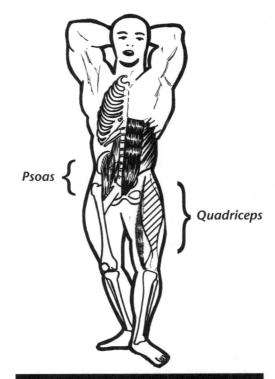

Psoas

Quadriceps

Figure 22 - The hip flexors

Figure 23
Front view - hip flexors (detail)

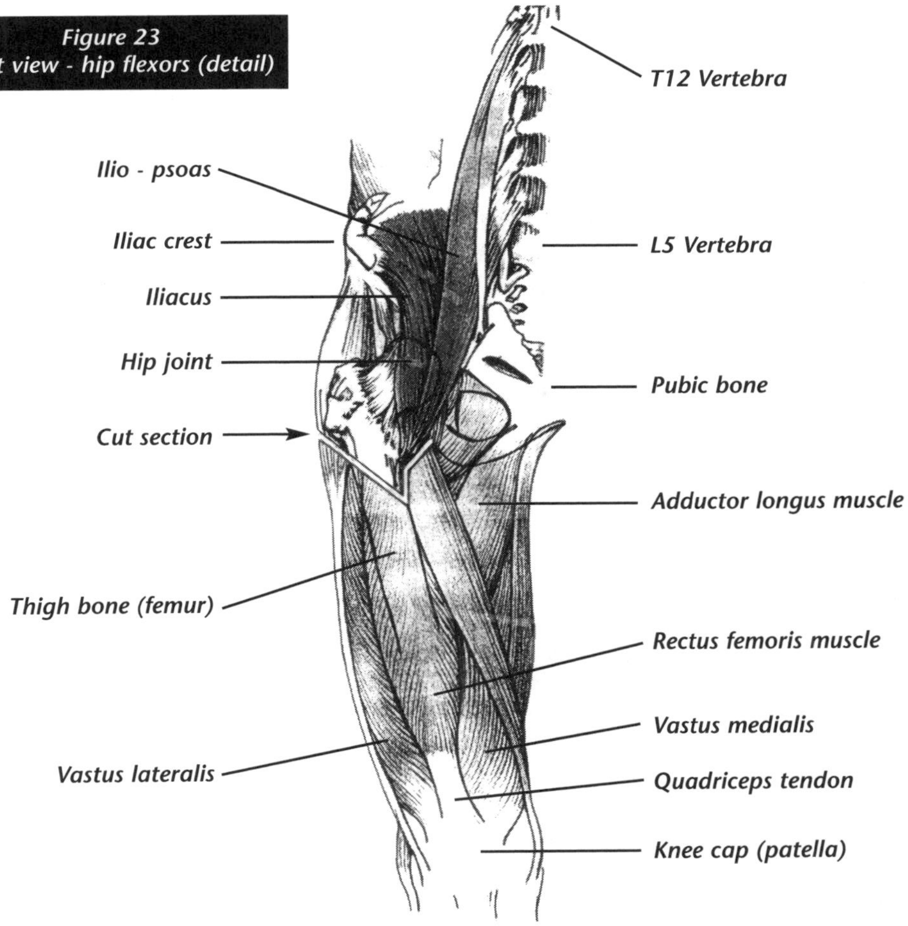

Ilio - psoas

Iliac crest

Iliacus

Hip joint

Cut section

Thigh bone (femur)

Vastus lateralis

T12 Vertebra

L5 Vertebra

Pubic bone

Adductor longus muscle

Rectus femoris muscle

Vastus medialis

Quadriceps tendon

Knee cap (patella)

In general, we can equate back pain to a lack of muscle strength in a corresponding section of the abdominal area and, in some cases, a combination of other tight muscle groups. The above is a generalisation and will vary from case to case. As we can see, certain imbalances are not visually noticeable and, although the posture appears normal, the effects are considerable.

As described above, a tightening of the quadriceps muscles can lead to an arching of the lower back. As this continues the lower back and psoas muscles also become contracted and the latter draws the lumbar vertebra forward. This creates stress on the spinal column and the discs in between. This pressure caused by a combination of tight back, psoas and quadriceps muscles can exert enough pressure on the spine to cause nerves to become 'squeezed' between the disc and the vertebra leading to the condition of sciatic pain.

From this common example above, it is important to recognise the fact that muscles work in conjunction with each other. A chain reaction can occur when misalignment of muscles in one part of the body causes the need for a compensation in another part, further up or down the line. In the above example, a further compensation for the hyperextension in the lower back (lumbar vertebra) could be a tendency to sway back at the knees.

IDENTIFYING PAIN

Injuries occur even in people who are fit or think they are fit. When an injury occurs, other muscles come into play to alleviate the pressure on the injured area. As a result, some of these muscles exert themselves more than they have done in the past. As they become stronger they, too, then tend to pull the body out of alignment further. So, once the injury has been resolved another problem has occurred which requires correcting. Muscle wastage (or atrophy) is common in sports and other injuries. Although the person thinks they are fit, they may still be in pain owing to increased pressure on the limbs or joints from other muscles that have been automatically recruited to keep the structure functioning as normally as possible.

While continuing to participate in sports where pain is still present in certain movements, it is necessary to first take appropriate action to determine what the pain is and employ clinical efforts (treatment, scans, etc) to alleviate the problem. If the pain still persists, before commencing an exercise program it is essential to:

1. Identify the area of pain - muscle, joint, tissue or bone
2. Assess the level of pain during the specific movements *(is pain only present when the activity takes place?)*
3. Determine the amount of restriction of the painful area
4. Determine whether the area has suffered a previous injury or trauma
5. Establish whether scar tissue is present which would restrict full range of motion?

Joint strains are a fairly common occurrence and can be corrected quite easily in the early stages. If there is any strain in any joint when exercising, it is important to:

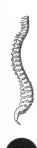

a) reduce the range of movement of the joint

b) if the strain persists, reduce the rotation of the joint (if externally or internally rotated at the joint)

c) if the strain is in a hinge joint (knee/elbow), reduce the extension or flexion at the hinge

d) if the strain is in the rotating joint and the hinge joint is hyperextended, bend the hinge joint to better engage the muscle between the rotating joint and the hinge joint e.g. single leg circle with the hand on the knee Exercise #22.

Neck strain during exercising can, in most cases, be alleviated by:

a) drawing the scapulae towards each other and then to the hip line without arching the back and

b) lengthening the neck (reducing any lordosis) Figure 24(b).

c) If the strain persists when exercising on your back, place a comfortable cushion under the head (not too high, as this will not help alleviate the condition). Keep the head rested during the exercise.

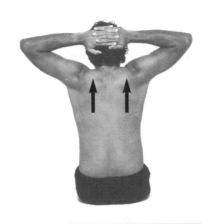

Figure 24(a) Incorrect

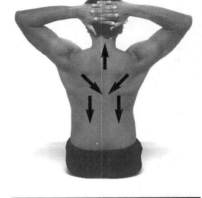

Figure 24(b) Correct

Lower back strain during exercising is generally caused by the back arching or hyperextending.

a) Flatten the back by imprinting the spine onto the floor and then B-Lining.
(If standing, imagine you are standing against a wall.)

b) If it is still arched, do some quadriceps stretches (See Stretches for Warming Up) to mobilise the hip joints, this may alleviate the problem almost immediately for a short period of time, but must be continued on a regular basis.

c) Tilt the pelvis under slightly (posterior tilt) to correct the arch. If lying down, do not lift the hips off the floor.

d) If lying down with the knees bent and the back is still arched, then draw the knees to the chest.

e) If standing, draw the rib cage to the imaginary wall, without rounding the shoulders, and bend the knees.

To summarise:
There are three areas, where, during the exercise routine, you should never feel any pressure, strain or pain:

i) The back
ii) The neck
iii) Any of the other joints.

Although the neck and back are also joints themselves, I have itemised them separately here for easier identification by those new to discovering their bodies through movement.

OVERSTRETCHING, OVERWORKING, OVERDOING IT. PAIN!!!

THE STRETCH AND WORK SCALES

When following an exercise or stretching routine it is important to listen to what your body is telling you.

The myth of 'NO PAIN, NO GAIN' is old fashioned and dangerous. The 'burn or pain' could actually be micro fibre tears of the muscle itself!

A certain amount of soreness is acceptable if you have not worked out for some time and decide to engage in even a mild circuit class. It is best, in these cases, to partake in a mild stretch class the next day to alleviate any aches and pains from the previous day.

Stretching muscles should be performed gradually and, if an uncomfortable level of pain occurs the next day, it may be an indication of excessive muscular work. Ease up on the regime and the situation should correct itself. Continual working and stretching through pain is not an intelligent approach to good body maintenance. The muscles need time to repair themselves before further exertion is applied to them. In the long term, this could lead to those niggling, recurring complaints that can haunt you for years! If you do have this problem, consult a trained, exercise oriented, health care professional or a qualified Pilates instructor.

Naturally, there is a certain amount of pain that occurs during training (even after proper warming up). In order to challenge ourselves to become better at any physical activity we intend to undertake, a certain pain level is acceptable. At what level is this pain acceptable is the real question? In any case, if the pain is sudden, sharp, uncomfortable or acute, it is our body telling us that we must cease that activity.

While performing the exercises, it may be useful to adopt the following Pain Scale guideline when assessing pain levels. This guide is in a very simple format and is intended to be used only to monitor 'normal' pain levels. If any unusual twinges or momentarily sharp pain occurs, reduce the exercise or stretch to a level that is comfortable.

The **Stretch Pain Scale** is a simple scale of 0 to 10. Zero being no stretch where no pain is felt and no stretch occurs.

Ten, on the other hand, is where the pain level is extremely uncomfortable and unbearable. The position cannot be maintained. This is a level where you feel there is no benefit to the movement or to your body. Regularly striving for this level may result in long term tissue damage and is to be avoided at all costs. (The only exception to this rule is the quadriceps stretch. See Exercise #11-13).

No stretch	mild stretch		strong stretch	stretch pain	'pain' pain

0.........................1.....2.....3.....4.....5..................6..........7.........8........................9.......................10

SAFE	WORK	DANGER

Figure 25

1-5 If you feel any pain or discomfort during a movement or stretch, ask yourself at what level this is. If it lies between 1 - 5 then you may feel a mild stretch and continued stretching in this zone is safe (taking into account that no other parts of the body are being affected).

6-8 If the 'strong stretch' is between levels 6 - 8, you will experience a strong muscular stretch but no pain. This stretch has a beneficial muscular feeling to it and you know that you are able to maintain the position comfortably. This has a 'doing you good' feel to it. You know you are really doing some work. You are being challenged at this level.

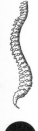

9 When approaching level 9, the feel of the stretch or movement changes from one of comfort to one of discomfort and pain. In this zone damage may occur. It is better to 'back off' to the work zone and continue the exercise than to risk forcing the muscles and possibly causing injury.

10 Level 10 is unbearable pain and should never be experienced.

Only very experienced athletes who understand their bodies through many years of training (and, usually, many injuries) would be able to continue working in what to us is the danger zone, and gain any benefit. The body awareness of athletes of this calibre is heightened, not only by the stringent demands they make on their bodies, but also by the mental discipline that their regimes require to attain the best result.

The **Work Scale**, on the other hand, involves muscular control. It, too, is on a scale of 0 to 10.

0   =   no work at all
1-5 =   the exercise can be easily controlled. Many repetitions can be performed at this level.
6-9 =   is an increasing challenge
10   =   the exercise cannot be controlled

The stretch/pain scale always dictates. What this means is that if the stretch/pain scale is 8 and the work scale is only 3, for that particular exercise, the 8 level is to be observed. Do not push the work scale to attain its challenge range (6-9). This will only push the stretch scale further! As the stretching routines continue on a regular basis, the stretch scale may ease back to 6 or so. In this case the work scale can then be increased to 4 or 5 and so on.

GRAPH I

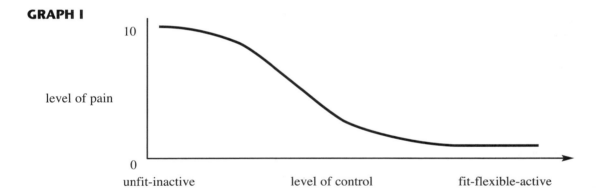

BODY POSITIONING FOR BETTER EXERCISING

Correct Posturing or positioning before commencing an exercise regime, or a specific exercise, is essential to connect the correct muscle groups. By assuming the correct posture, energy is focused on the muscles that require it and not wasted in other areas or unnecessary movements.

This is especially true when beginning an exercise that is totally new to your body. New exercise programs generally require more concentration and control to which the body may never have been subjected.

For instance, take triathletes who never attempted a yoga class before. The new positions require a great deal of thought and focus. Muscles are being subjected to new positions and forcing these movements can cause injury, especially as they are held for some time. Such athletes may not spend an hour stretching. It is always important to keep in mind that any new routine for the body must be approached with caution.

Because triathletes are quite fit compared to the general population, they also approach physical challenges more readily and sometimes do throw themselves into new regimes, with the mental attitude that their bodies can endure any new venture.

The muscles, however, have memorised only certain movements as a result of countless hours of repeating those movements over many years. Once the body, and mind, have approached a routine in a certain manner it is difficult to change that pattern without changes to the result. These changes may initially be adverse, such as slower times or not jumping as far, until the muscles accept their new regime as the 'set' basis upon which to progress.

Our bodies will invariably take the easy way out. They will perform movements that require less effort and concentration. When we are not focused, our bodies will cheat on us! For example, lie on your back with your arms extended to the ceiling above your chest. This may be done with or without hand weights. Make sure your arms are not above the face or neck, but directly above the chest in line with the shoulders. Keeping the arms in line with the shoulders, slowly open the arm out to the sides (floor) and close to the ceiling again. Repeat this half a dozen times. Notice that as you do more, the arms slowly start to move above the face when in the air and in line with the head when open to the floor. This has the effect of the shoulders being gradually raised with the neck muscle engaged. Imagine the effect when the exercise is repeated hundreds of times!

To work specific muscles groups requires concentration and effort. To maintain an almost perfect regime of such movements, until they form the required engram so the movement becomes automatic, requires a pattern for muscular development and achievement for that movement.

For this to be accomplished, a routine needs to be established. Once this is achieved, then any new movements to the body, such as the athlete attempting yoga, can be approached safely. The participant can perform their own 'self-check' as to the requirements, benefits, limits and dangers to which their bodies will be exposed.

ESTABLISHING A PATTERN FOR MUSCULAR CONTROL

We have developed a formula in the search to perform an exercise to the best of one's physical ability, no matter what level of fitness you are.

When the formula is followed it may at first seem difficult to approach all the points at the same time. However, by systematically covering each aspect sequentially, and maintaining that principle before the next is undertaken, would be an ideal way of perfecting the exercise and developing good technique.

The formula, P/A/P, B, B, E, E, Q, has been designed to make each exercise precise and to gain the most benefit out of each movement or series of movements. A gradual approach to new routines will establish a solid foundation to use as a springboard to developing the movement or routine for greater speed, range or control.

It has been found that if this formula is adhered to, it is almost impossible to perform a routine incorrectly, or for an instructor to devise an incorrect movement for their client.

1. POSTURE/ALIGNMENT/POSITION

When commencing an exercise it is important to ensure that the correct position or alignment for the exercise is established. If this is not correct from the start, the movement can become sloppy and less effective. Especially in regard to rehabilitation exercise programs. Establishing and maintaining the correct position of a limb, the pelvis or torso is important to the final outcome. A difference of one centimetre in an exercise can mean a difference of 10, 20, 30, 40 or even 50% in the effectiveness of the exercise. Imagine a gymnast on the parallel bars or on the beam who moves one centimetre off their projected alignment. They may lose control, balance and even worse, fall off the apparatus. Or a tennis player who misses the 'sweet spot' on the racquet more times than his opponent. It could mean the difference between winning and losing, between perfection and 'close enough is good enough' or developing the type of body you really want.

Training the brain to search for these small differences requires assistance. The help of a mirror can identify major differences in position and alignment.

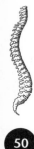

Some questions regarding this principle of the formula are:

1. Are the hips square?   **2.** Is the leg in line with the shoulder?   **3.** Is the torso upright?
4. Is the foot flexed?   **5.** Are the shoulders level?   **6.** Is the back straight?
7. Is the stomach flat?   **8.** Is the neck elongated?   **9.** Are the shoulders relaxed?
- And so on.

2. BACK

Ensure that the back is in the required position for the start of the exercise. Generally, when lying supine, the back should be as flat as possible, B-Line and zip up. These help to maintain a firm centre.

What do we mean by zipping up the B-Line? Imagine you are trying to get into a very tight pair of jeans. Many of us have tried this before. We either lie on the bed or floor or bend ourselves over double to pull our stomachs in! Well, imagine the same now. The lower abdominals are B-Lined prior to starting the movement of the zipper. We then have to keep B-Lining as the zipper is closed all the way up and imagine the B-Line coming up with the zipper.

For many, this may be one of the few times we actually feel our lower abdominals contracting! This attempted, continual connection helps to strengthen this group of abdominal muscles. It is also these lower abdominals that greatly assist in the relief of lower back pain and in the ability to tuck the pelvis under.

Control of the rib cage also provides stability for the spine (see section below: Breathing). When upright, is the back straight or is there a lean to one side? Is the lower back arched or the upper back too rounded? Is the head tilted forward or backward?

All these can be corrected to a certain extent by realignment and re-education of the muscles. If the problem is more structural, as in some cases of osteoporosis, the spine and back should be aligned in as best a position as possible, without causing any discomfort.

3. BREATHING

The breathing has been covered in another section under the same title. However, the manner of instruction for the breathing is important.

In many instances when performing challenging small movements, many people hold their breath. It is generally accepted that one should breathe out on the effort. What exactly is the effort is open to debate. For example, take a body building exercise when lying on the back on a low bench, holding on to a heavy weight and working the triceps. Extending both arms above the head and returning them to the vertical position performs this movement. We can notice several 'faults' with this action.

This movement is usually done with the feet on the ground, creating an arch in the lower back before the exercise has even begun. This, in itself, can cause stress to the lower back and certainly a tightening of those muscles. When extending the arms overhead to the floor, the back is arched even further as the pectorials almost 'lock' past a certain point. Limited mobility occurs at the shoulder joint. The breathing is usually a short breath in as the arms extend above the head and, as they are drawn back to the starting position, a heavy blow out occurs with a great deal of straining of the entire torso.

Would we perform the same triceps exercise for a tennis player wishing to improve their serve or overhead smash? We hope not. The example above may be suitable for those who require short bulky muscles, although the breathing technique leaves a lot to be desired from a stamina-improvement point of view. More elongation is required for the tennis player. The weight would be less, the back would be flatter (feet on the bench) and the arms would need to be lengthened more.

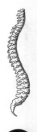

To control the exercise and work on the specific muscle group in a more focused manner, other areas of stress and strain should be eliminated as much as possible. The breathing is usually one of these stress points. If the body builder were to breathe as calmly as possible and still perform the exercise in whatever manner they wished, it would all look too easy; they may need to lighten the weight to gain more control. The breathing would change their ability to perform the movement as they were used to doing previously. To those around them they would not appear to be working hard at all.

However, if the tennis player, with calmer breathing, a flatter back and less facial expression were to perform the same exercise with the same weight as the body builder and with more ease - everyone would wonder what sort of super athlete this were displaying such control and ease of movement.

Breathing has an important role in allowing the body to improve its ability to cope with stress, whether mental or physical. Often the instruction is given as, ' Lift your leg and breath out.' The message the mind has received is, 'Move the limb and, at the completion of the movement, breathe out.'

In an exercise routine, the breathing instruction should ideally be, 'Breathe in (or out) <u>as you</u>....'. Breathe for the duration of the movement to reduce stresses and strains, which if correctly accomplished can avoid injury incurred through lack of concentration during the movement. If you run out of breath, then the body begins to strain as the breath is held and the movement continues to be performed.

Breathe calmly in through the nose and sigh out of the mouth.

As the breathing becomes the norm for the movement, the movement can be increased to faster repetitions, still breathing in normally for 2, 3 or 4 repetitions and out for the next 2, 3 or 4. Controlled, calm breathing can certainly lead to an increase in physical performance.

4. EXERCISE

The exercise is now performed as perfectly as possible. If you are unable to perfect the exercise with the correct breathing in the first half a dozen movements, do not despair. Practice the exercise with whatever breathing feels comfortable at the time. Get the body to move and understand what is required of it. As this becomes more feasible and familiar, then adjust the breathing to the correct requirements.

Even when performing advanced exercises, return to the basic versions every so often. You will find that, they too, can be difficult to perform as more focus and connection is applied to the simpler movements.

5. ELONGATION

Exercises performed with continual lengthening of the muscle group being worked tend to have several distinct advantages. The benefits gained from muscle *lengthening* can be:

• leaner muscles, less 'bulk'   • increased mobility of the joint
• reduced stress on the joint   • reduced 'clicking' of the joint
• increased awareness of specific, isolated muscle movement

Lengthening the muscle should, of necessity, require the muscle group to initially be stable and injury free. Lengthening of injured muscles can place more load on the fibres and lead to further problems.

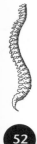

In many exercise routines, especially those involving heavy weights, it is noticeable that the movement of the limb through its full range is not usually achieved. The body does this to reduce the amount of stress on the joint. However, not extending the muscle through its full range has the effect of shortening that muscle. In biceps curls, when lifting a heavy weight, the arm is rarely extended close to its full length. The upper body is also usually curled forward in order to prepare it to take the strain of the next lift. This movement, when the weight touches the thigh, has the illusion that the arm has performed a close to full extension.

If the exercise were to be performed correctly through full range with the same amount of effort, the weight would need to be reduced as the strength in the biceps muscle fibre, when almost fully extended, is not as great. Once greater strength is achieved in the extended position, then an increased weight can be safely applied.

Similarly, in the abdominal curl, if the knees are bent at an acute angle at the knee joint (heels too close to the bottom), the exercise has less chance of achieving length in the abdominals. The forward contraction has the effect of squashing the abdominals. This makes them bulge upwards rather than scoop. The exercise then becomes strained and ineffective.

With the knee joint at a right angle (feet further away from the bottom), better performance can be noticed with increased effect on the muscle worked as long as the abdominals are scooped in. With the knee joint at greater than a right angle (obtuse angle), the hip flexors are more elongated and, ensuring that the lower back remains flat on the floor and B-Lining, the exercise is more challenging. If the 'pull' of the hip flexors of the thigh are further reduced, the abdominals will work more effectively (see PAC with cushion under the knees, Exercise # 25).

Strength in length would be the epitome of muscle tone for almost every athlete. Female classical ballet dancers find that they are extremely flexible but not strong enough in their extreme ranges of movement. To them this is a weakness. Even to look at a weight while exercising would, to them, have the effect of bulking the muscle! However desirable the strength factor is to them, they would not be seen dead in a weight training gym!

On the other hand, triathletes would welcome more flexibility without compromising their strength. But they would never be seen dead in a ballet class! Correct body usage with the technique in this book can lead to both groups being catered for. Dancers can, with the correct use of weights, gain greater strength without fear of bulking their muscles. Triathletes can improve their flexibility without compromising their strength or speed. In fact, both could benefit from the one common factor - reduced risk of injury.

Elongation during the entire movement, through full range and during all repetitions requires concentration and effort. As the muscle tires, the first thing to happen is the reduction in the lengthening of the muscle. The muscle can work more easily in a more contracted position. When this happens, stop the exercise. Only continue when you are able to maintain an elongated 'line' to continually enhance, and strive for, the lean, long (and strong) look.

6. QUESTIONS

After all of the above 5 principles of the formula have been systematically performed, eventually in the space of five seconds or less, the final and most important part of the equation remains.

It is a check list of all of the above, and more. Besides mentally assessing and correcting each movement, the exercise may still not be performed correctly. This is shown in several ways and the following question would cover and correct the movement by returning to the formula:

Where do you feel the exercise working?

This should be in muscle groups for that movement alone. E.g. when exercising the legs or lower limbs, the shoulders should not be hunching or straining. There are many areas where things can go wrong. The rule is - if it feels uncomfortable or hurts, don't do it!

Common sense should dictate at all times. Some of the most common areas to focus on are listed below. This is by no means an exhaustive list. As a guide, it would, optimistically, introduce an understanding of correct and safe muscle movement. This would then install a greater sense of awareness of the moving body and encourage you to listen to your body when it talks to you.

A simpler way of visualizing the movement of the limb is to concentrate on the movement of the bone itself and not the muscle. This way, better control without strain may be more possible to achieve.

THE FUNDAMENTALS OF BODY AWARENESS AND ESTABLISHING CORRECT EXERCISE POSTURE

Getting to know your body is an important start to the Pilates Method or, indeed to any exercise program. As people develop physically, they also develop physical habits. Some of these may have taken years to develop, such as lifting objects in a certain way. Whatever the reason, just as in one of the laws of physics, our bodies prefer to move along the path of least resistance when performing any task. That path of least resistance is accommodated by our subconscious. It is stored into our memory banks for future reference for the same, or similar, movements. Our bodies will automatically want to cheat on us when we perform many of life's everyday movements.

Many of these movements may be incorrect. Such as walking with our feet pronated. This may explain why some people get headaches and others may get lower back pain. However, we are not aware that this could be the cause of some of these symptoms. Understanding and correcting the smallest of imbalances, or incorrect positioning, of our bodies may eliminate many of the minor, or major, aches and pains we become so accustomed to living with.

By becoming more aware of your body, and the space within which it moves, is an important factor in understanding more about your physical being. By mentally identifying and 'feeling' individual parts of your body without having to move those parts may be difficult to attain at first. However, when this can be achieved, understanding how to move correctly becomes an easier process. The result is that our physical and mental reflexes become more heightened; we can judge distances better, control the amount of effort we apply to physical tasks and even relieve physical stress and mental anxiety.

Understanding our body also means listening to it when it adversely reacts to situations. Not to push it when, mentally, we think we can perform a task, but physically we have slight doubts. As you develop your body with this program you will begin to realize that without correct mental focus, the movements become sloppy and ineffective. Mentally you also feel the same. It is important to realize that when your body has performed several repetitions of a movement as correctly as possible, and the extra one is not up to standard, then do not continue with the remaining repetitions. One perfectly executed movement is worth any number of sloppy ones!

There are several phrases that you will come across in this book. These key phrases shall be repeated often. They are essential to the basic control of the exercise and the achievement of beneficial results.

When you think you have gone as far as you can - EXTEND IT!

When moving the limbs or any part of the body, a greater feeling of working all muscles, especially the unused, smaller ones is achieved by lengthening through the movement. For example, when standing or lying on your back, B-Line and keep the ribs lengthened away from the hips while also pressing the shoulder blades to the hips. This requires more abdominal contraction and helps to keep the spine long, alleviate pressure on the vertebrae and discs and helps to keep the spine more flexible.

When working the arms or legs and these limbs require lengthening, do not lock the knee or elbow joints. This can cause stress on that joint. If these joints are hyperextended, then the bones are merely being locked together and the muscles will strain rather than work. With these hinge joints, it is best to keep them unlocked, not bent. Too much of a bend will not allow the muscle to lengthen and restrict mobility of the limb from the socket. With the joint unlocked it is still possible to lengthen out of the socket (without moving the hip or shoulder) to attain the mobility required.

FEET - STANDING

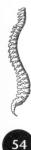

When standing, imagine that each of your feet are like tripods (See: Tripods Page 43). Maintaining this equal loading while moving the rest of the body will feel as if you are anchored to the floor. In this way, a key element of good posture is achieved. Work the abdominals as described below, keeping the legs straight, but not locked. The ribs are lifted from the hips in a vertical line, B-Line, relax the shoulders to the hips and lengthen the neck.

FOOT POSITIONS

The feet are an integral part of the exercise. Not to be regarded as attachments at the end of our legs, the feet are also continuously working. There is no time that they are flopping around and left unattended.

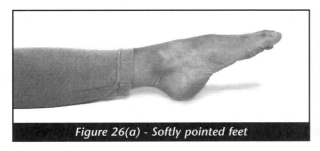
Figure 26(a) - Softly pointed feet

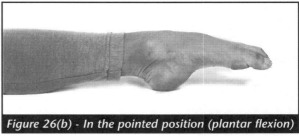
Figure 26(b) - In the pointed position (plantar flexion)

In the pointed position (Figure 26(b)) the feet are pointed where the joint between the big toe and the second toe are in line with the centre of the knee cap. This line of strength prevents the foot from either inversion (turning in) or eversion (turning out). The stretch should be felt on the top of the foot and a lengthening sensation should be achieved rather than a cramped pointing of the toes. Attempting to overstretch through the toes can result in a cramping of the arches of the feet. If this occurs, 'softly point' the feet (Figure 26(a)).

To achieve the flexed position (Figure 28) or dorsi flexion, press through the heel as far as possible. This should draw the toes towards your knees without curling them back. If the toes do tend to curl back, draw the balls of your foot towards you. This may take some practice. If, when flexing the feet, the calves feel excessively tight, stretch them before continuing with the rest of the program.

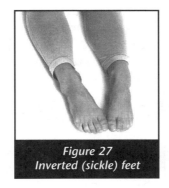
Figure 27
Inverted (sickle) feet

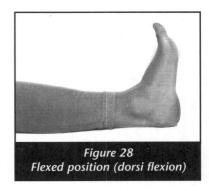
Figure 28
Flexed position (dorsi flexion)

The position for feet flexed and turned out and pointed and turned out are clearly shown in the photographs below. When turning out, imagine the muscles of the inner thigh doing the work for this movement, rather than forcing the rotation from the knees or the feet (Figures 29 (a) and (b)).

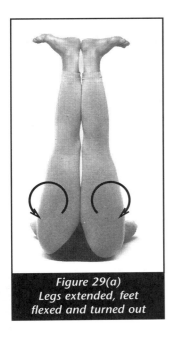
Figure 29(a)
Legs extended, feet flexed and turned out

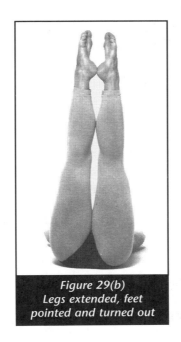
Figure 29(b)
Legs extended, feet pointed and turned out

IF YOU ARE NOT TONING IT, YOU'RE FLABBING IT!

For the majority of women, the flabby muscle areas that they would desperately wish to tone are:

1. the back of the arms   **2.** the section of abdominals below the navel
3. the buttocks   **4.** the outside of the hips and
5. the back of the thighs

For men it is principally the entire abdominal section.

If we could keep the muscle toned continually, fatty deposits would have less chance of accumulating in these areas. For example, how often do we find fatty deposits on the front of the thighs? As we are continuously walking, climbing stairs, jogging or running, the quadriceps muscles rarely have a chance to rest in our everyday routines. We do not have to worry about toning this group.

Especially when it comes to the buttocks, it is not often that this group is continually held firm in our normal, daily routines. Hence, the muscle becomes slack and requires extra work to reshape it to an acceptable size or shape. Gripping the buttocks is not essential to maintaining good tone and may, ultimately, produce more bulk. When standing, keeping them pinched is preferable.

To firm this muscle group (the gluteus maximus), imagine sitting in a chair with a coin being held just inside the cheeks of the buttocks. Stand up out of the chair without dropping the coin and then keep the buttocks pinched as above. Do you notice how, automatically, the gluteals want to release and all the effort transfers to the quadriceps? This may take some practice to realize how to hold the gluteals on a regular basis. Perform this pinching of the buttocks whenever you are standing or sitting. This will reduce the need to use heavy, unnecessary exercise routines that can build bulk and create tighter, lower back muscles.

THE CENTRE

The abdominals are there to provide support for the back in its function of keeping the body erect. It also assists in rotation of the torso.

This is easily tested by the following: allow your stomach muscles to go slack. Notice what happens to your posture. It begins to slump. The shoulders move forward and down

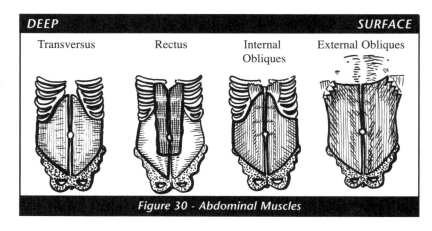

Figure 30 - Abdominal Muscles

and the body becomes shorter. This can also lead to reduced breathing capacity as the lungs become squashed. Now sit upright on your sit bones without arching the back. Notice that at once your stomach pulls in towards your spine. The lower back muscles also engage to straighten the back. This also has the effect of, not only making you sit taller, but also supporting the back and 'lifting' pressure off the back.

Another way of describing this is to sit as though you are lifting your ribs vertically away from your hips, without allowing your ribs to move forward or the shoulders to hunch. If we can keep the length between the ribs and the hips and then B-Line, I am certain that up to 30% of all back problems could be more easily solved. This positioning of the spine is similar to alleviating the pressure off the vertebrae and discs by 'separating' them from each other. This in turn can take some of the pressure off any nerves that are being impinged. If this position can be maintained while the body is in motion, not only will the posture improve, but mobility in the spine would increase.

SUPINE POSITION - LYING ON YOUR BACK

Place a mat on the floor and lie down on your back, feet extended and together and hands relaxed by your sides. You will observe that there is an arch in the lower back (Fig.31(a)). If this position is too uncomfortable, bend

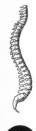

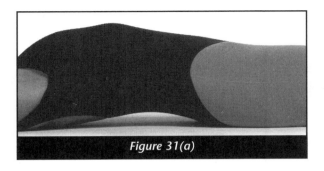

Figure 31(a)

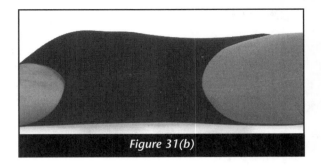

Figure 31(b)

both legs very slightly. Place you hand in the space between your back and the floor and B-Line. Can you feel the abdominal muscles engage? (Do not push you feet on the floor or tilt your pelvis up to the ceiling).

Remove the hand and continue to B-Line. Can you feel how much deeper you are now working from the abdominal area? You may even feel as if the back itself is pressing to the floor (Figure 31(b)). This is one method of identifying and feeling your 'centre'. It is the area from which all controlled strength and flowing movement emanate.

By B-Lining we also engage the mid and upper abdominal sections. It is far easier for most people to engage the mid and upper abdominal sections without any connection in the lower abdominals!

It is a common error to feel that if the back is not flat on the floor then the back is not 'flat'. The attempt here is to keep the back supported while the spine is in a normal, or neutral, position. This is where the hips are neither tilted in a tuck nor extended to arch the back.

THE NECK

When lying on your back do not allow the neck to arch as this will tighten the neck muscles and jut the chin forward. Lengthen the back of the neck to stretch these muscles and improve thoracic/cervical postural muscles

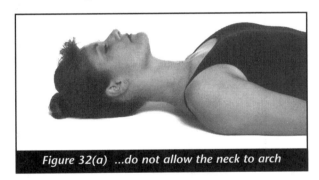

Figure 32(a) ...do not allow the neck to arch

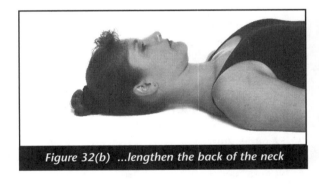

Figure 32(b) ...lengthen the back of the neck

SITTING

Similarly, in a sitting position, most people will have the tendancy to slump (Figure 33(b)). When sitting lift up out of the hips or sit tall on your sit bones. Imagine your spine is similar to a rod. Perfectly upright, at right angles to the floor and running from the base of your spine through the crown of your head. Now imagine that your torso is sliding up that rod while your hips remain anchored to the ground, B-Line, shoulders relaxed to the floor (Figure 33(a)).

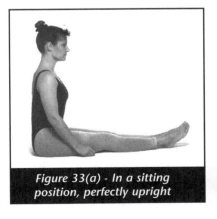

Figure 33(a) - In a sitting position, perfectly upright

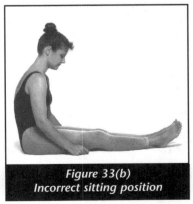

Figure 33(b) Incorrect sitting position

The Complete Guide to the Pilates Method

SHOULDERS

Neck and shoulder tension is a common problem with most people, whether they exercise or not. This tension is caused by the trapezius muscles. Often when we are encountered with a sudden shock or surprise our arms, shoulders and neck immediately tense in an almost defensive reaction. When we lift objects, even such as holding a baby on the hip, we hunch the shoulders. When our friends give us a neck or shoulder rub they comment on how these muscles are 'as hard as rocks'.

This tension can be created from situations as far afield as sitting in front of a typewriter or computer all day, to worrying about the results of an exam! This tension shortens the muscle group, as tension does with any of the muscles, which hunches (and slightly rounds) the shoulders and arches the neck.
To reverse this process sit in an upright position and start by feeling the tension in the neck and shoulder muscles with your fingers. While gently applying pressure to the shoulder muscles, hunch your shoulders. Now gently allow the shoulders to release by pressing the shoulder-blades to the floor as hard as you can while growing your spine to the ceiling. At the same time slightly squeeze the shoulder-blades

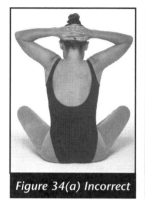 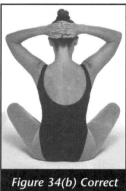

Figure 34(a) Incorrect   Figure 34(b) Correct

together. This has the effect of opening the chest and allowing a slight release of the pectoral muscles that round the shoulders forward. This may even cause some discomfort between the shoulderblades as the muscles stretch. Repeat this movement several times and feel the tension release further each time.

Other methods of feeling the tension release is to:

1. Place your hands on the top of your head, with your elbows forward. (If you place your elbows wide open, the trapezius muscle remains in a contracted position.)
2. Sit with your arms extended away from the body at shoulder height, lengthening through your fingertips.

You may feel your neck and shoulders already tense. Hunch them up as much as you can. Do you notice that the chin also tends to jut forward.

Now focus on:

1. Pressing the shoulder-blades to the floor as hard as you can with a deep sigh out
2. Lengthen further through the fingertips
3. Grow as tall as you can out of your hips
4. Slightly squeeze the shoulder-blades together without creating further tension in the back (Figure 35).

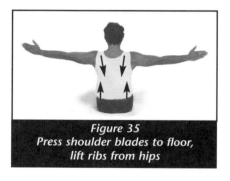

Figure 35
Press shoulder blades to floor,
lift ribs from hips

Repeat the movement by hunching only 10% as much as before. Now perform the release proceedure above and hold it for 20 seconds while breathing normally. Repeat four more times and then rest your hands by your sides. Do you feel taller? More relaxed? Does your body feel lighter? Do you mentally feel more relaxed?
By contracting the opposite muscles to the ones that automatically create the tension, positive muscle control negates the effects of, not only the physical, but also the mental tension.

NECK

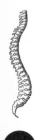

Tension in the neck (and shoulders) can lead to poor posture and severe headaches. Tight trapezius and cervical muscles make the chin jut forward and create an arch in the neck. To create positive muscle control, press the shoulders to the floor and slowly draw the tip of the chin slightly down towards the rib cage while lengthening the crown of the head to the ceiling. Can you feel the stretch in the back of the neck? This feeling may even extend down the upper back towards the shoulder blades. Do not squash the chin to the chest.

IMPRINTING

As the spine is a major focal point of movement for
the rest of the body it is important to keep it supple
and strong. The movement of the spine when
getting up off a floor or lying down should
resemble that of leaving an imprint of the spine
in soft sand. When lowering or raising the torso
to or from the floor each vertebra should be moved
one at a time, without any sharp or jerky
movements. It may facilitate how to achieve this
by some analogies:

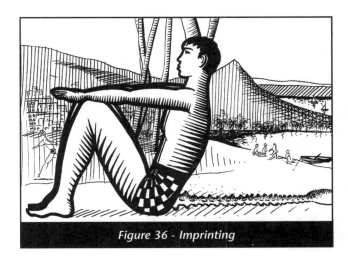

Figure 36 - Imprinting

1. Imagine the spine is like a string of pearls
   being lowered (or raised) one at a time or

2. As if your spine is stuck to a wheel;
   as the wheel smoothly turns, so does each
   vertebra move one at a time.

In a sitting position when curling the spine up or down, more flexibility in the back can be achieved by reaching
forward through the fingertips while rounding the back.

The Complete Guide to the Pilates Method

NOTES

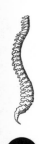

There are only three things in life that will help us to live longer.
"Strength and suppleness together - and a good sense of humour"
Anonymous

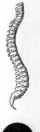

CHAPTER 4

STRETCH, STRENGTHEN AND RELIEF IN THE SAME MOVEMENT. THE EXERCISES THAT WILL CHANGE YOUR LIFE

Although we are promoting isolation of muscles to attain a leaner, longer body with control and precision of movement, we should keep in mind that the body works as a whole. When attempting to isolate a particular muscle for a stretch, other muscles may come into play.

It is true that the toe bone is connected to the cheek bone via a complex arrangement of tissue, muscles, connecting joints and mental perception.

Case Study

While attempting a normal hamstring stretch with the back in an upright position and holding onto the bench, the patient felt a cramping of the muscles in the mid back area just below the shoulder blades. The cause of this was that, in the attempt to increase the forward lean and, thereby, increase the stretch for the hamstring, the latissimus dorsi and lower trapezium gripped. The client was found to also be tightening the muscles between the shoulderblades (the rhomboids). This was easily corrected by depressing the shoulders and slightly rounding the upper back. The pain disappeared and the effectiveness of the hamstring stretch was maintained.

WARM UP AND STRETCHING BEFORE YOUR PILATES PROGRAM

Stretching is an all important part of warming up the muscles before any physical activity. It 'wakes up' the muscles by providing an infusion of blood and nutrients into the more open tissue. Because of the increased pliability of the muscle, more flexibility is achieved and the underlying joint is also able to move more freely. There are two main types of Stretches - Dynamic (involving motion) and Static (no motion occurring).

The following Sensible Stretching Techniques should be followed when performing stretches.

1. Stretch the muscle gradually

2. If any joint pain occurs, reduce the pressure on the joint by
    a) reducing the angle at the joint (e.g. seated hamstring stretch - if more pain is felt behind the knee joint than in the hamstring, bend the knee until more hamstring stretch is felt)
    b) control the rotation of the joint e.g. when performing side splits and pressure is felt in the knee joint, this may be because the femur is internally rotated. Externally rotate the thigh until only the adductor is felt
    c) if joint pain still occurs, do not continue

3. Do not stretch injured or torn muscles

4. If you have achieved maximum range of movement and do not feel the stretch, continue the movement as a means of mobilizing the joint and loosening up before working the muscle

5. If stretching a group of muscles affects another group (e.g. a thoracic stretch strains the shoulder joint) do not continue without further guidance

6. After the muscle has been worked, stretch all muscle groups
    a) to reduce bulking of the muscle
    b) to reduce the risk of injury to joints, muscles and tendons
    c) to reduced post exercise soreness in the muscle
    d) to maintain and increase joint mobility
    e) as part of your cool down and also
    f) to increase flexibility

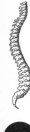

When starting any exercise routine it is necessary to limber up before launching into the 'meat' of the program. This can generally take the form of a 5 minute bike ride, a jog around the block or EFFECTIVE STRETCHING that gradually lengthens and mobilizes the muscle groups for longer than 90 seconds at a time.

Gentle stretching can also form a part of this warm-up for those incapable, or those who find it uncomfortable, to engage in the former methods of warming up. This category can include those with injuries. Stretching and strengthening the uninjured muscle groups, by isolating them, is an ideal means of 'staying in shape' for those with any injury. As long as there are no effects on the injured muscles, tendons, joints or ligaments, or the area immediately surrounding the injury, exercises contained here can keep the body 'toned' and 'functioning' rather that not doing any exercise for the body at all.

To substitute this 'extended' stretching in place of a warm-up routine, for the average person, is not detrimental to the end result of the program. It is, in some cases, more beneficial and safer, than some warm-up routines that are currently performed.

If the weather is cold, or if you feel excessively 'tight' in the muscles, then extra time should be spent on stretching. As to the time of day when one should stretch; this is entirely up to the individual. Some of us feel much better stretching in the early morning (to 'wake' ourselves up) and others feel as if they are unable to move at all until the end of the working day, when the body has been mobilized and looser, to accommodate any physical activity.

There is no evidence to suggest that using 'extended' stretching techniques is detrimental to physical achievement, when performing a controlled, non-strenuous exercise program. In fact, in the majority of cases using the Pilates Method, participants have frequently reported that they felt more energized, more flexible and less mentally and physically stressed at the end of their routines.

In order for the muscle to achieve its maximum range of movement, a continual stretch into the specific muscle area is required. Combined with the correct breathing technique, (in through the nose for 5 seconds, sigh out of the mouth for 5 seconds without depressing the chest) helps to increase blood flow to the muscles being stretched. This helps a great deal in improving the elasticity of the muscle as well as in the elimination of lactic acid from the muscle group.

The 'START STRETCH ROUTINE' described at the beginning of the program is intended to stretch isolated muscle groups. The ideal order for stretching the body is to start with the back (lower and upper) and shoulders, the hamstrings, and then the quadriceps. An interdependence sometimes exists between some muscle groups and may reduce the primary intention of the stretch. For example, tight calves may reduce the intended stretch for the hamstrings. Therefore, it would be prudent to stretch the calves first before continuing with a hamstring stretch.

POINTERS FOR SAFE EXERCISING:

1. If at any time a stretch or exercise feels uncomfortable or painful, reduce the intensity of the stretch or exercise by reducing the range of movement or ease the pressure off the joint.

2. If sharp pain or referred pain to another part of the body occurs, stop the exercise. Seek the advice of a qualified Pilates Instructor on the movements you are doing (eg. when performing back or neck extension).

3. If a movement feels too easy, first follow the principles and formula to enhance the quality of the movement, then increase the intensity of the exercise by progressing to the next version of the movement.

4. If you ever feel your neck straining during a supine exercise, support it with cushions or pillows. The exercise may then be completed without any strain on the breathing or on muscles that are not the 'working ones'.

5. Whenever performing an exercise that requires you to be on your back, B-Line and flatten the back (without tilting the pelvis), unless otherwise stated. As the exercise progresses and you feel that your back is arching it may mean one of several things:

    a) The leg position is too far away from the centre. Draw the knees closer to the chest or bring the legs more vertically into the air

    b) If the position requires the head and shoulders to be contracted forward (shoulder blades just off the floor, ribs to hips in the same plane), this contraction may slowly be releasing as the exercise progresses. Attempt to maintain the contraction at all times

    c) The abdominal muscles are gradually weakening and the back muscles are beginning to take over. If the back comes off the floor even one millimeter, (if you can slide a ruler between your back and the floor), then the back may be doing more work than the abdominals. Stop the exercise. There is no point in continuing the exercise if the powerhouse of the anatomy (the abdominals) is no longer controlling the movement.

6. Challenge yourself! Progress can only be achieved by increasing the intensity, or range of movement, of the exercise by a few percentages each time. Follow the program as close as you can and you will gain more confidence and body awareness. You will feel a different person!

THE STRUCTURE OF THE EXERCISE PROGRAM

1. PREREQUISITE EXERCISES

Certain intermediate or advanced exercises require basic strengthening or stretching of muscles in order to perform that exercise comfortably and safely. These prerequisite exercises will be described at the beginning of the exercise section of the book.

2. PURPOSE OF THE EXERCISE/MUSCLES WORKED

Muscles that are to be worked are described here. In many instances where exercise routines are described, an explanation as to an association with a 'non exercise' movement is provided.

This is where we can see the use of what is being achieved in the routine and how those muscles need to function outside an exercise situation.

3. DESCRIPTION OF THE EXERCISE AND CORRECT BREATHING

The description of the exercise
  • Start position (P/A/P)
  • Back position (B)
  • Breathing (B)
  • Exercise (E)

4. KEY POINTS

These are major mental or physical points to consider when doing the movement. These slight movements, though possibly obvious or minor in their application, produce a considerable difference in the effectiveness of the execution of the exercise. Remember, even a centimeter difference in the movement of a particular position can mean up to 50% difference in the effectiveness of the exercise!

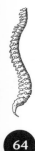

5. CARE NOTES (Q)

At the end of the description of each exercise are CARE notes. These notes are the most commonly encountered problems that may arise during the movement and how to counteract these stresses safely. They would answer the majority of questions that would be asked regarding major points about the exercise.

6. REPETITIONS

The ideal number of sets and repetitions of each exercise are suggested. Remember, the end of each repetition is the continual motion of the following repetition until the final one is complete. Do not rest in between each repetition as the muscle will relax and need to be reconnected for the next repetition. One movement flows into the next while maintaining muscle tone and consistency of deep breathing and muscle identification through isolation. Thus, mental and physical stamina and endurance are improved with the resultant enhancement in confidence in what the body is able to achieve.

Only complete the number of repetitions with which you are most comfortable. If you can only manage 6 repetitions before you start to feel that the exercise is not 'working properly' or effectively, then stop after 6.

Add one repetition each week until the required number is achieved. I have mentioned 6 repetitions as this is more than 50% of the generally required amount. By completing more than 50%, you are closer to finishing and the psychological half way barrier is passed.

NOTES

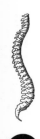

CHAPTER 5

"Contrology® is complete coordination of the body, mind and spirit. Through Contrology® you first purposefully acquire complete control of your own body and then through proper repetition of it's exercises you gradually and progressively acquire that natural rhythm and coordination associated with all your subconscious activities." - J.Pilates

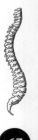

CHAPTER 5 - THE COMPLETE PROGRAMS

The following programs have been designed with careful thought to the ability of the person undertaking the routines. If any of the exercises are too difficult, please follow the instructions in the Chapter under Safe Exercising (Page 63).

At the end of the exercise section, I have included suggested programs for daily routines from the four sections. Each week add an extra exercise from the section until you are able to complete all the exercise comfortably, then move on to the next section.

The programs are gradually more challenging. If the participant feels that any exercise from one section is too difficult, he/she may substitute that exercise from a previous section without a drastic overhaul of the entire section. Therefore, exercises may be chopped and changed to accommodate the participant's requirements. You may tailor make your own program until you are able to follow the routines suggested here.

1. The Routine for Lower Back Pain and Weak Abdominals.
   For those who have MINOR lower back pain that does not involve referred pain (down the legs, etc.) and for those with weak abdominals.

2. The Basic Routine. For those starting an exercise program.

3. The Intermediate Routine. For those who have no back pain and are of a reasonable to average fitness level.

4. The Advanced Routine. For those who can complete the Intermediate Routine with ease, exercise regularly and require a challenge.

Remember - please seek medical approval or advice from a qualified Pilates practitioner, before embarking on any exercise program, especially if you have never attempted these exercises before.

I apologize, in advance, for the length of explanation in some of the exercises. If, at the start, you cannot understand it all to make full use of it, do not worry. Start with only two or three of the instructions for each exercise. As these become understood and engaged, then add another instruction. I feel that by giving you all the knowledge, you can use what you require until such a time as you can use it all. This not only provides you with the most comprehensive set of instructions ever written for the Pilates exercises, but will also answer all your questions in relation to the exercises.

You should wear snug, but comfortable clothing. If possible, place a mirror next to you so you can see yourself in order to correct any postural deviations that you would not otherwise notice. It would be ideal to have a friend read out the instructions to you, once you have a mental picture of what the exercise looks like from the photos or diagrams. For all the floor routines, use a thick but firm mat to lie on.

When embarking on the program try to commit yourself to it for at least three times a week for six to eight weeks. The first two weeks will be the toughest. Any good, effective exercise program takes time to establish itself within your muscle memory. It took years to create the body you now have - it is not going to change overnight with the Pilates Method. Stick to it and you will gradually start to see changes, not immediately, but in the long term.
You will be glad you persevered. Good Luck!

PS. I have included a 'notes' section for you at the end of most of the exercises. Use this area to take notes on 'revelations' that you may have for future reference.

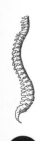

EXERCISE # 1
REST POSITION

1. This position can be used at any time during the program.

2. PURPOSE: It is a great way to relax and allow the spine to stretch.

3. EXERCISE: Starting position: Kneel back on your haunches, with your toes extended.

   i) Keeping your buttocks on the heels as much as possible, slowly Breathe Out and curl the spine forward while sliding your fingers on the floor ahead of you.

   ii) Stretch all the way forward through your fingertips, while pressing your shoulder blades to your hips. Forehead rested on the floor. Breathe In without moving.

   iii) Relax in this position.

4. KEY POINTS: On every breath out press the buttocks onto your heels and lengthen your chest to your knees. This is a very small movement. When you feel you have lengthened as far as you can, relax in this position. After several breaths, attempt a further small lengthening movement.

5. CARE: If there is any discomfort in the knees, place a cushion behind the knees. This will keep the buttocks off the heels, but will allow for a more comfortable stretch.

REPETITIONS: One set of 10 BI (Breaths In) and 10 BO (Breaths Out)

BREATHING: Breathe in and out deeply and slowly for 10 breaths.

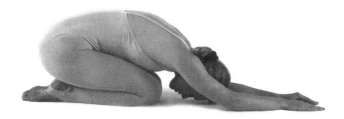

NOTES

THE WARM-UP

EXERCISE #2
STANDING SPINE ROLL

1. This is a basic prerequisite for all exercises.

2. **PURPOSE:** Loosens up the spine, hamstrings and lower back.

3. **EXERCISE: Starting Position:** Stand as tall as you can with your feet apart shoulder distance.
    Feet parallel. Imagine your spine is stuck to a wall. B-Line, pelvis slightly tucked under (posterior tilt),
    shoulders relaxed.

    i) Bend your knees slightly and Breathe Out deeply as you slowly and sequentially peel your vertebrae off
    the wall one at a time by lowering your chin forward to your rib cage, then ribs to hips while pressing your
    lower back into the imaginary wall.

    ii) Half way down, take a deep breath in and then with another deep breath out relax the body as far as it
    will comfortably go, keeping the knees bent. If you cannot touch your toes, do not force yourself to do so.
    At the bottom of the movement take a deep breath into the chest, keeping the B-Line.

    iii) Breathe Out and return to the standing position by reversing the movement, imprinting your spine onto
    the imaginary wall, or imagine stacking your vertebrae one on top of the other. Start the movement by
    tucking the pelvis and drawing the hips to the rib cage, engage the lower abdominals, then pressing the
    middle and upper abdominal to the spinal wall. This movement should be felt in the anterior portion of the
    body (abdominals).

4. **KEY POINTS**: Keep the body weight over the tripods of the feet.
    Lengthen the ribs from the hips on the upward roll. Flatten the stomach,
    relax the shoulders.

5. **CARE:** If the back feels the slightest strain in doing any of the work on the
    upward roll, bend the knees until only the abdominals are doing the work.
    Do not force yourself to touch you toes if you are unable to do so comfortably.

6. **REPETITIONS:** ONE SET OF 10

    ADVANCED: Do the movement with the legs straighter at each attempt.

    BREATHING: BREATHE OUT (BO) ON WAY DOWN, BREATHE IN (BI)
    at the point of flexion (relaxation) and breathe out on the way up.

NOTES

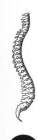

EXERCISE # 3
THE START STRETCHES

1. This is a basic prerequisite exercise for the whole program.

2. **PURPOSE** Stretches the lower and middle back, opens the groin area.

3. **EXERCISE: Starting Position:** Sitting upright on the sit bones as if against a wall, with knees drawn towards the groin and dropped open, soles of the feet together. Ensure that the lower 15 centimetres at the base of the back is perfectly erect at all times. If it is not, place the feet further away from the groin or sit up against a wall and allow the spine to touch it without leaning against it at any time. The body should not be slumped into the hips. Sit as tall on the **sit bones** as possible.

i) Reach the arms to the ceiling, stretching the spine; bend the elbows and place the fingers down the back between the shoulder blades. Imagine that you have suction cups on your finger tips, so as you curl forward the hands do not slide up towards the neck. This will increase the intensity of the stretch. Keep the shoulders relaxed when lifting the ribs from the hips.

ii) Breathe Out as you CURL THE HEAD FORWARD onto the chest and down towards the rib cage LETTING THE UPPER SPINE FOLLOW. You are attempting to roll your nose towards your B-Line, keeping the lower 15cms of the spine as **upright as possible**. LET THE CHEST RISE AND FALL WITH THE BREATHING. If this is difficult because of the compression of the chest in this position, breathe into the back (See: BREATHING, page 33). Press the knees open to the floor.

iii) Hold the position for the breath in, without moving, then curl further forward towards the B-Line on the next breath out. Curl as far in to the B-Line as possible on the first movement. After this the movements are very small, if at all.

This movement is very slight and can be felt quit strongly in the muscles on either side of the spine, in the lower back or across the shoulder blades.

4. **KEY POINTS:**

  1. Perpendicular lumbar spine, lift out of hips without hunching the shoulders,
  2. B-Line, elbows close to and behind the ears,
  3. Relax Shoulders and neck, curve from rib cage.
  4. Sit tall on sit bones at all times.
  5. Press the knees open to the floor to open the groin. If this is uncomfortable, keep the knees relaxed open. If the feet are too close to the groin, you may feel as if you are rolling back onto the hips. Place the feet further away from the body until you are sitting tall comfortably (unsupported by the hands). Do not allow the body to lean forward so the head moves over the feet. This means a lean from the hips rather than a bend at the rib cage, changing the muscles required to be stretched. On the breath in, do not allow the body to move at all.
  6. DO NOT CROSS THE HANDS TO AVOID ANY STRAIN ON THE NECK WHEN CONTRACTING FORWARD

5. **CARE:** If you feel the shoulders hunch or the neck strain, relax the shoulders.
Keep the shoulder blades to the hips. Do not force the chin onto the chest, roll it comfortably down to the rib cage, and then nose to the B-Line.

6. **REPETITIONS:** Ten breaths in and ten out, one set.

7. **BREATHING:** Breathe In, allow the chest to expand through all areas, especially sides and back.
IF BREATHING IS DIFFICULT BREATHE 'INTO THE BACK' or do not contract forward too far.

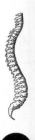

VARIATIONS:

ALL SITTING TALL ON SIT BONES, B-LINING. REPEAT THE EXERCISE AS ABOVE MOVING THE FEET TO THE DIFFERENT POSITIONS DESCRIBED BELOW FOR THE TEN BREATH REPETITION.

EXERCISE # 4

BOTH LEGS STRAIGHT AND TOGETHER IN FRONT, FEET POINTED. MAKE SURE KNEES ARE POINTING UP TO THE CEILING SO THE THIGHS ARE NOT TURNED OUT. PRESS ANKLE BONES TOGETHER. IF THE FEELING IS TOO STRONG BEHIND THE KNEES, BEND THE KNEES only slightly.

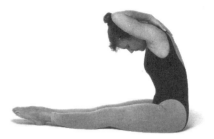

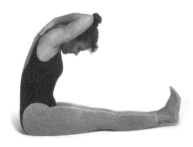

EXERCISE # 5

BOTH LEGS STRAIGHT AND TOGETHER IN FRONT, FEET FLEXED PRESSING THROUGH THE HEELS. This should be felt comfortably in the spine and mild to strongly in the hamstrings.

EXERCISE # 6

LEFT LEG STRAIGHT IN FRONT OF THE LEFT HIP, FOOT FLEXED, RIGHT LEG BENT AT THE KNEE WITH THE SOLE OF FOOT AGAINST INSIDE OF THE LEFT KNEE OF THE EXTENDED LEG.
HIPS SQUARE Leg in line with the hip. Do not adjust the hips to establish the position, ONLY ADJUST THE LEGS.

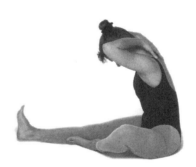

EXERCISE # 6A

REVERSE LEGS AS IN #6).

DURATION:
10 SLOW BREATHS IN AND OUT, CONTRACT FURTHER FORWARD ON THE BREATH OUT.

NOTES

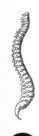

The Complete Guide to the Pilates Method

EXERCISE # 7
SPIRAL STRETCH

1. **PREREQUISITE:** TO BE ABLE TO CORRECTLY PERFORM UPPER BACK STRETCHES, SHOWING NO PROBLEMS or strain IN THE BACK whatsoever. Do not perform this stretch if you have any back problems or back pain.

2. **PURPOSE:** To stretch the sides between the armpit and the hips, lower back muscles and shoulder joints.

3. **DESCRIPTION: Starting Position:** Sitting as in Exercise # 6.
   Breathe in and take both arms reaching for the ceiling (left leg straight, right leg bent).

   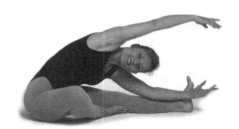

   i) B-Line and Rotate the torso to the right, rotating the centre of the Breastbone (sternum) past the point of the bent knee.
   ii) Breathe out and stretch the torso sideways along the extended leg. Hold onto the foot or the ankle of the straight leg with the left hand.
   iii) Breathe in without moving, **Breathe out** and bend the left elbow to try to lengthen the left armpit towards the left knee (without bending the knee) and the right hand past the left foot and parallel to the floor. **Breathe in**, without moving. Repeat 10 times.
   iv) To finish, lengthen BOTH ARMS past the extended foot, REACHING OUT OF THE HIPS to the ceiling (remaining rotated) then rotate back to the front position. Relax the hands by the sides. Change sides.

4. **KEY POINTS:** HIPS SQUARE, B-LINE, BOTH SIT BONES ON FLOOR, LENGTHEN THROUGH THE SPINE, UPPERMOST SHOULDER TO CEILING, NO OVERARCHING IN LOWER BACK. TRY TO MAINTAIN THE TOP ARM/ELBOW BEHIND THE TOP EAR. The more rotation that can be achieved, the better the stretch.

5. **CARE:** If the rotation feels uncomfortable in any part of the body - stop.
   Keep the body directly over the extended leg and slightly in front of it for a better stretch.

6. **REPETITIONS:** 10 BI and 10 BO. One set each side.

BREATHING: BREATH IN as you hold the position; BREATHE OUT as you stretch over extended leg.

VARIATIONS:
If you are flexible enough to hold the foot of the extended leg with the top hand, do so. Place the other hand on the floor INSIDE the extended leg. When Breathing Out, bend the elbow of the top hand to the ceiling holding onto the foot for leverage, and walk the fingers of the bottom hand along the floor to stretch that side.
ON EVERY BREATH OUT ROTATE AND LENGTHEN THE TORSO FURTHER.
Press the hips of the bent leg into the floor for a better stretch. B-Line, especially on the breath in.

NOTES

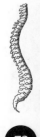

EXERCISE # 8 - 1
CALF STRETCHES

1. **PREREQUISITES:** Nil

2. **PURPOSE:** To stretch, and strengthen, the calf muscles (gastrocnemius and soleus).

3. **EXERCISE: Start Position:**
   Stand with the balls of the feet on the edge of a step. Place a tennis ball between the ankles to prevent the feet from rolling outwards on the rise. Place a thick pad between the knee to prevent the knees from rolling in and help to connect the inner thigh muscles.

   i) B-Line with a slight tuck of the pelvis. Breathe In and rise up onto the balls of the feet as high as possible. Do not drop the tennis ball.

   Think of working the muscles in the feet rather than working from the calves.

   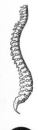

   ii) Breathe Out as the feet lower to below the level of the step, pressing the heels down as far as possible. As the heels lower below horizontal, squeeze the pad and lightly turnout the upper thighs. The knees and upper thighs have a tendancy to roll in at this point.

4. **KEY POINTS:** Do not drop the ball nor the pad.
   If the knees are too wide apart, use a thicker pad.
   The point of the rise should be on the ball of the foot between the big toe and the second toe. This should be in alignment with the centre of the knee cap.

5. **CARE:** Do not allow the lower back to arch at any time. Tuck, if required to prevent this.
   Do not drop into the heels; lower and press down gradually.

6. **REPETITIONS:** 15-20 reps

NOTES

The Complete Guide to the Pilates Method

EXERCISE # 8 - 2
ALTERNATING CALF STRETCHES

1. **PREREQUISITE:** Exercise # 8 - 1

2. **PURPOSE:** To stretch the calves more then the previous exercise, especially if one calf is tighter than the other

3. **EXERCISE: Starting Position:**
   Stand on the edge of a step on the balls of the feet.
   B-Line and **Breathing In**, rise up onto the balls of the feet as high as possible, imagine holding a tennis ball between the ankles.

   i) Breathe Out as the right heel lowers below the level of the step, while the left leg stays high on the ball of the foot, bending the knee.

   Slightly turnout the right thigh to prevent the knee from rolling in.

   ii) Breathe In as you rise up on the right foot only to the height of the left foot.
   Change feet and repeat with the left foot.

   Only use the muscles of one foot at a time.
   Do not let the hips swing out to the sides by sinking into them.

4. **KEY POINTS**: As in Exercise # 8 -1

5. **CARE NOTES:** As in Exercise # 8 -1

6. **REPETITIONS:** 20 reps alternating legs

Variation for the soleus: As the heel lowers below the horizontal, bend the knee to stretch the soleus.

NOTES

EXERCISE # 9 - 1
HAMSTRING STRETCH - BASIC

1. This is a basic prerequisite exercise.

2. **PURPOSE:** This exercise is to safely stretch the hamstring muscles for those with extremely tight hamstrings or with back pain.

3. **EXERCISE: Starting Position:**
   Lie on your back with knees bent (right angle at the knee joint).

   i) Bend one knee to the chest and place a long towel or IsoToner around the heel.

   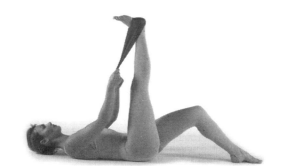

   ii) Slowly extend the heel to the ceiling. Keep extending the foot until a strong stretch is felt in the hamstring (not behind the knee). If the leg fully extends and there is no effect on the spine, move on to the Normal Hamstring stretch (Exercise #9-2).

   iii) Breathe In holding the position. Take a **DEEP Breath Out** and press the heel to the ceiling for more stretch,without the tailbone lifting off the mat.

4. **KEY POINTS:** B-Line and keep the hips firmly pressed to the floor without arching the back. Place a cushion under head if the neck arches. Do not hunch the shoulders or allow them to come off the mat.

5. **CARE:** B-Line, shoulder blades slightly squeezed together, neck long.

6. **REPETITIONS:** 10 Breaths In and 10 Breaths Out. Change legs. Two sets on each leg alternating. It is important to alternate the legs rather than do all 20 repetitions without stopping. This gives the muscle some 'breathing space' before subjecting it to more stretching. By doing this we do not 'push' the muscle to its limits without a break. More benefit is derived as a better conscious stretch is achieved during the second set.

BREATHING: BO press through the heel. BI hold the position.

ADVANCED: As this becomes easier, slowly straighten the bent leg. Continue to draw the leg being stretched towards the same shoulder, without bending the knee. As the stretched leg is able to maintain a straight position, gradually extend the leg on the mat to an almost straight position, without the back arching, foot flexed.

NOTES

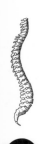

EXERCISE # 9 - 2
HAMSTRING STRETCH - II

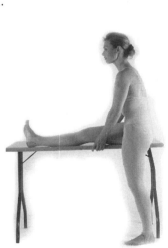

1. **PREREQUISITE:** Stretched calves.

2. **PURPOSE:** To perform a more specific stretch on the hamstring group.

3. **EXERCISE: Starting Position:** Standing upright, place the right foot on a chair or table, with the leg extended up to hip level. If you are more flexible, the leg can be raised higher. Left foot facing forward.

    i) Hips square and parallel, foot flexed and knee cap pointed to the ceiling. B-Line.
    ii) Keep the knee as straight as possible. B-Line and Breathe Out as you lean your chest forward. Imagine that on every breath out, you are growing taller as you lean forward out of the hips. DO NOT BEND THE HEAD OR CHEST TO THE KNEE.
    Look upright at all times without tilting the head to the ceiling
    iii) Hold the position for the Breath In; Breathe Out, lift and lean forward further (only a slight movement is required).

4. **KEY POINTS:** If more pressure is felt behind the knee than in the hamstring, bend the knee. Imagine someone is lifting you out of your lower back, lift up and away from the tailbone, almost as if you are attempting to arch the very lower part of the back. If performed correctly, this stretch should be immediate and quite strong.

5. **KEY POINTS:** Keep the pelvis square and level to the floor. Keep the supporting leg firmly planted into the floor at all times directly below the hip. Flex the foot as much as possible to achieve more stretch. B-Line.

6. **CARE:** If any extreme stretch occurs in any part of the back do Exercise # 8.
    If there is tightness between the shoulder blades, round the shoulders slightly.
    If there is a mild tightness in the lower back (from lifting out of the hips) bend very slightly from the lower back until the discomfort eases.
    HIPS SQUARE, HIPS LEVEL, SUPPORTING LEG DIRECTLY UNDER THE HIP, KNEE NOT HYPER-EXTENDED, UPPER BACK STRAIGHT, LEANING FORWARD FROM THE HIP JOINT.
    If too much pressure is felt behind the knee, bend the knee. You should feel only the hamstring.

BREATHING: BREATHE IN LENGTHEN SPINE TO THE CEILING, BREATHE OUT OPENING CHEST TO THE WALL IN FRONT. REMAIN IN THIS POSTURE FOR 10 BREATHS. ON EACH OUT BREATH EXTEND FURTHER UP AND FORWARD TO FEEL THE STRETCH.

VARIATIONS: EXERCISE # 10
    a) Sit on one leg on a flat bench. This position is easier to keep the hips level. The leg on the ground is bent and the toe is facing forward. This is easier than the version above.
    b) Standing, (as in #9-2) take the leg at a higher level than the hip. This may begin to lift this hip, so place the hand of the same side to press the hip to the floor.
    This movement alone will create the start of the stretch.
    c) Use the arms to lean the body further forward by holding on to the leg or the bench and bending at the elbows.

NOTES

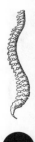

EXERCISE # 11
HIP FLEXOR STRETCH I - PRONE

1. This is a basic prerequisite exercise for those who cannot do Hip Flexor Stretch II or III.

2. **PURPOSE:** To stretch the quadriceps muscle group, especially for those with knee joint problems.

3. **EXERCISE: Starting Position:**
   Lie on a mat face down with a small, folded towel placed under the stomach to assist the B-Line.
   Bend the right leg drawing the foot to the buttock. Reach back with the right hand and grasp the foot.
   The body should remain in a straight line, without the shoulders twisting or the knee shifting away from the
   straight line with the hip. A mild to strong stretch should be felt along the front of the right thigh.

   i) Breathe Out and bend the right elbow in order to bring the heel closer to the buttock, B-Lining and
   pressing the right hip bone to the floor. Hold the position for the breath in and repeat 10 times, drawing
   the heel closer to the buttock each time, while B-Lining more. This should be an extremely strong stretch
   in the middle of the thigh. Press the right hip bone into the floor.

4. **KEY POINTS**: The towel is to help prevent the back from arching and taking any pressure. If the hip bone
   is flat on the floor, then progress to Hip Flexor Stretch II, as long as there are no knee joint problems that
   may arise from putting pressure on one knee.

5. **CARE:** If you cannot bend the knee to the buttock comfortably, it is a clear indication that the quadriceps
   are, indeed, tight. If any pressure is felt in the back, it may be arching too much, or the body is not in
   a straight line, then place a towel around the foot, hold on to the towel and draw the foot towards the
   buttock. Ensure the foot is in a direct line with the buttock and drawn over to the inside of the thigh.

6. **REPETITIONS:**
   2 sets of 10 breaths, alternating

   BREATHING:
   10 breaths in and 10 breaths out in each set.

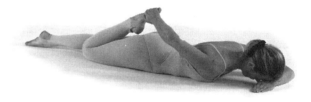

NOTES

The Complete Guide to the Pilates Method

EXERCISE # 12
HIP FLEXOR STRETCH II - STANDING

1. **PREREQUISITE:** This is a basic prerequisite exercise.

2. **PURPOSE:** To stretch the thighs, to connect the B-Line and open the lower back.

3. **EXERCISE: Starting Position:**
   To stretch the left thigh, stand with the right leg on the floor and the left leg bent
   on a chair or holding on to the left foot with the left hand. Some balance may be
   required. This balance improves over time as more stretches are completed.

   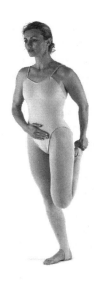

   i) Breathe Out as you tuck the pelvis under. This can be greatly assisted by
   'pressing' the left buttock to the floor and drawing the pubic bone to the navel
   with the assistance of the right hand.

   ii) Breathe In, hold the position. **Breathe Out** and tuck under more.

4. **KEY POINTS:** Remain leaning slightly forward all the time.
   This 'opens' the lower back and the continual tuck opens it even further.

   Ensure that the hips are level and square before starting the exercise. The bent leg
   usually has a tendency to lift the hip on that side. By simply squaring the pelvis
   (parallel to the floor) a mild to strong stretch may be felt.

   Ensure that the front of the thighs are level with each other. If the thigh being stretched is forward of the
   (other) supporting leg, press the knee down to the floor as much as possible while bringing it in line with
   the supporting leg, without arching the back. This should induce a stronger stretch with a small movement
   of the thigh downwards.

5. **CARE:** This stretch should be felt very strongly on the quadriceps only (middle to top of the thigh) and
   no other place. (This 'pain' level may exceed the 9 level). When the stretch stops, so should the pain.
   If the pain continues after the stretch has stopped, do not repeat.
   Sigh on the breath out, relax the shoulders.

6. **REPETITIONS:** 2 sets of 10 BI and 10 BO, alternating legs.

BREATHING: Breath in without moving, Breathe out on the tuck.

NOTES

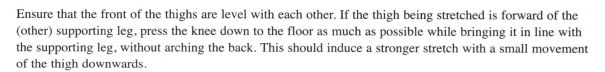

EXERCISE # 13
HIP FLEXOR STRETCH III - KNEELING

1. **PREREQUISITE:** Achieving Hip Flexor II Stretch without feeling much stretch.

2. **PURPOSE:** To stretch the hip flexors, iliopsoas; connect the B-Line and open the lower back.

3. **EXERCISE: Starting Position:**
   To stretch the right thigh, place a thick towel or a piece of dense foam under the right knee, with the foot up against a wall or on a chair. If this is uncomfortable on the front of the foot, place a soft pad under the foot. This position is easiest achieved by placing the hands on the floor and then putting the knee/leg into position. Bend the left knee and place both hands on the left knee and come into the upright position.

   i) The exercise now follows the same description as Hip Flexor Stretch II, Exercise # 12.

   ii) Place the right hand on the right buttock and the left hand just above the pubic bone.
   Press the buttock to the floor and draw the pubic bone to the navel.

4. **KEY POINTS:** It is important to make sure that the hips are not 'thrust' forward as this can arch the spine and put pressure in the lower back. The movement of tucking the pelvis under is hardly perceptible, but can be very strong. Do not release the stretch until the full ten breaths in and out are completed.
   B-Line! This will assist in a stronger stretch.
   Ensure the foot of the supporting left leg is at right angles to the knee so no undue pressure is place on the toes of the foot. Use the Tripod for this foot.
   More stretch can be achieved by placing some mild pressure with the hands to enhance the tuck, as the muscles may be too tight to achieve this on their own.
   To achieve a greater stretch imagine the hip bone of the leg being stretched, drawing strongly up to the rib cage on that side. Visually there will be no difference in the movement, but a deeper, stronger stretch can be achieved in this manner.

5. **CARE:** Same as Hip Flexor Stretch II, plus after stretching each leg, place the hands on the floor to change legs.
   The closer the knee to the wall, the better the stretch.
   If there is any pain in the knee joint, stop the exercise and try Exercise # 11.
   Keep the hand on the buttock only - not in the lower back.

6. **REPETITIONS:** 2 sets of 10 BI and 10 BO, alternating legs

BREATHING: 10 BI and 10 BO. Hold the position on the breath in, tuck the pelvis on the breath out.

ADVANCED VERSIONS:

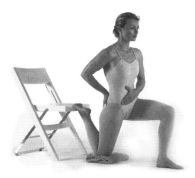

   If minimal stretch is felt with the above exercise then:
1. Place the supporting leg further forward and lean the entire body forward away from the wall and heel. Still, without arching the back, tuck the pelvis in this position. The stretch will be felt higher up the quadriceps towards the hip bone.
2. If 1. above is too easy, stay in the forward leaning position, reach back and grasp the foot away from the wall towards the buttock. Try to maintain the tuck without arching the back. This should induce an extremely strong stretch towards the top of the thigh.

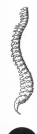

THE BASIC ROUTINE FOR LOWER BACK PAIN & WEAK ABDOMINALS

EXERCISE # 14
ONE LEG LIFTS - SUPINE

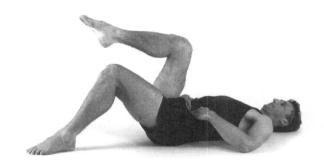

1. **PREREQUISITE:** Warm-up stretches.

2. **PURPOSE:** Basic Abdominal connection for the lower abdominals.

3. **EXERCISE: Starting Position:**
   Lie on you back (supine) with the knees bent at 45°.
   Without tucking, **B-Line** and place your fingers
   on the insides of the hip bones. Press firmly.

   i) Breathing out, draw the right knee towards your chest without the right buttock lifting off the ground.
   Do not place any pressure with the left foot on the floor.
   As the foot is lifted off the floor you may feel the abdominals push up against the fingers.
   Draw the abdominals in as hard as you can away from the fingers.

   ii) Hold the leg towards you for the **Breath In**, then **Breathe Out** as the leg is slowly lowered to the floor.

4. **KEY POINTS:** Sigh on the breath out and flatten the rib cage to the floor.

5. **CARE NOTES:** If the lower back continues to arch when the leg lifts, place the non moving leg up on a chair.

6. **REPETITIONS:** 10 on each leg, alternating after each repetition.

   ADVANCED:
   Attempt the same abdominal connection while either

   i) extending one leg on the ground
   ii) drawing both knees to the chest at the same
   time without allowing the back to arch.

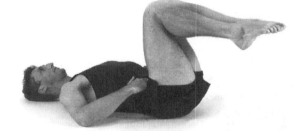

NOTES

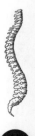

EXERCISE # 15
SLIDING LEG

1. **PREREQUISITE:** Warm up stretches.

2. **PURPOSE:** Maintaining abdominal connection when the body is lengthening.

3. **EXERCISE: Starting Position:** Lie on your back with legs extended and fingers placed on the lower abdominals. Press firmly. Draw these muscles in from the fingers. **B-Line**.

   i) Breathing out, bend one leg up to your chest, slowly sliding the foot along the floor, intensifying the control from the lower abdominal muscles.

   ii) Breathe In as the leg slowly extends away STILL drawing the abdominals away from your fingers.

4. **KEY POINTS:** Imagine the abdominal muscles are 'connected' to the thigh and that they are drawing in tighter as you draw the leg towards you. As the leg extends away from you let the abdominals lengthen and flatten.

5. **CARE NOTES:** Do not tighten the buttocks. On the breaths in and out draw the ribs to the hips, breathing into the shoulderblades. Keep the neck lengthened and the shoulders relaxed.
   If the neck is arched place a small cushion under the head.

6. **REPETITIONS:** 10 on each leg, alternating after each repetition.

VARIATIONS:

1. **MORE CHALLENGING:** Start with the right arm on the floor above the head. Breathe In as the right leg draws towards you while raising the right arm to the ceiling. Extend both the arm and the leg to the floor while B-Lining and flattening the rib cage to the hips.

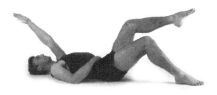

2. **EVEN MORE CHALLENGING:** Repeat Variation 1 while using both arms and both legs together, trying to control any arch in the back by B-Lining and flattening the rib cage on the breath out (extension of the body).

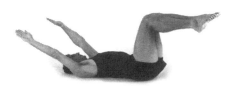

NOTES

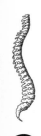

The Complete Guide to the Pilates Method

REST POSITION WITH KNEES TO CHEST FOR EXERCISES LYING ON THE BACK

Lie on your back on a comfortable mat. Draw the knees to the chest and place the hands on the ankles, drawing the heels into the tailbone without lifting the buttocks. Lengthen the neck and press the shoulder blades to the hips. This is the standard position for the start of most exercises which then progress to a contraction position (head forward, shoulder blades off the ground, arms forward past the hips).

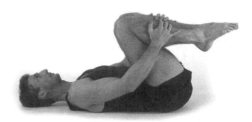

POSITION WITH CUSHIONS FOR ALL EXERCISES

Lie on a large cushion or several pillows where the shoulderblades are at the junction of the floor and the cushion. There should be no gap between the back and the floor at any time during the exercise, especially if the arms are raised into the air or behind the head. The head, neck and chin should be comfortable, with at least a golf ball space between the chin and the chest at all times. The eyes should be focused at a point slightly above the knees if the knees were raised vertically.

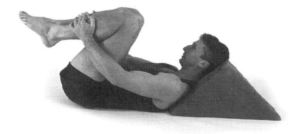

EXERCISE # 16
PREPARATION - WITH CUSHIONS

1. **PREREQUISITES:** Warm up stretches

2. **PURPOSE:** To strengthen, gain control and feel the entire abdominal section working.

3. **EXERCISE:** Starting Position:
   Lying on the cushion, draw the knees to the chest and
   hold on to them lightly with your hands.

   i) Breathe Out as you extend the hands forward past
   the hips and just off the floor, while extending the legs
   vertically into the air.

   ii) B-Line and draw the ribs to the hips.

   iii) Breathe In as you return to the start position.

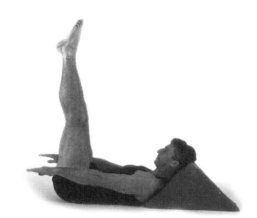

4. **KEY POINTS:** Keep the eyes focused above the knees.
   Deep sigh out. B-Line hard to connect the
   abdominals while scooping them for greater effect
   and support for the lower back.

5. **CARE NOTES:** Only raise the legs as high as you can to where the back does not arch at all.
   As you complete more repetitions the abdominals may weaken and the back take over.
   Stop at this point.

6. **REPETITIONS:** 10 reps. Rest for half a second between each repetition to gain continual tone in the muscle.
   Eventually, do not rest at all.

NOTES

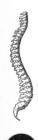

The Complete Guide to the Pilates Method

EXERCISE # 17
PREPARATION

1. **PREREQUISITE:** Warm up stretches

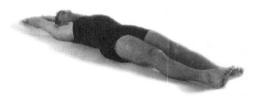

Figure i

2. **PURPOSE:** Abdominal work to control and reduce overarching in the lower back.

3. **EXERCISE:** Starting Position:
   Lie supine on the floor with arms above the head and legs together, toes pointed (Figure i)

   i) Breathe In as you raise the arms to the ceiling and bend the knees sliding the toes on the ground (Figure ii)

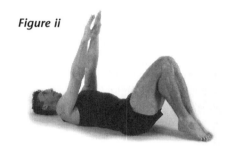

Figure ii

   ii) B-Line and Breathe Out as you:

   i) contract forward, extending the arms past the hips just off the floor and

   ii) raise the legs vertically (Figure iii)

   iii) Breathe In as you raise the arms vertically and bend the knees so the toes touch the floor

   iv) Breathe Out as you extend the arms and legs to the floor to the start position.

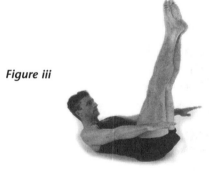

Figure iii

4. **KEY POINTS:** Stretch through the fingertips; slide the toes along the floor keeping the heels off; keep the shoulders pressed to the hips at all times.

5. **CARE NOTES:** Do not jerk up, keep the rhythm smooth during the movement. If the neck starts to strain after several movements use cushions under the head and only take the arms back as far as is comfortable.

6. **REPETITIONS:** 10 reps

NOTES

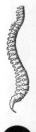

EXERCISE # 18
THE HUNDREDS - BASIC

1 **PREREQUISITE:** Start Stretches.

2 **PURPOSE:** To strengthen the abdominal group of muscles.

3 **EXERCISE:** Starting Position:
Lie on your back with knees to your chest, hands relaxed on the ankles.

i) B-Line and Breathe Out as you contract forward. Extended the hands forward through the fingertips, palms down, 15 cm off the floor.

ii) Raise your legs vertically into the air, flexing your feet and externally rotating your legs from the thighs. Touch the back of the knees together to stretch the hamstrings and connect the adductors (this will take the pressure off the front of the thighs) Pinch the buttocks slightly.

iii) Keeping the eyes on the knees and **B-Lining, Breathe In** for five seconds and **Breathe Out** for five seconds. Repeat 10 breaths in and out without resting. (The ten seconds in and out by 10 repetitions equals 100, hence, the name Hundred).

4. **KEY POINTS:** Keep the rib cage drawn to the hips at all times, shoulder blades off the mat and relaxed forward, eyes on the knees.
If the shoulders drop back on the breath in, contract forward further on the breath IN.
Scoop the abdominals.

5. **CARE:** If the back arches or strains, turn the legs in and bend the knees slightly.
When the knees are bent keep the heels in a vertical line with the buttocks to keep the back flat.
If you feel the neck strain, place a cushion under the head, raise the head on each BO, rest on the BI remembering to keep the B-Line even in the rest position. As the neck becomes stronger, raise the head up for 2 breaths, and so on.

To assist the B-Line, place a small weight on the lower abdominals and draw the abdominals away from the weight, especially on the breath in. When the weight no longer moves, remove it.

6. **REPETITIONS:** 2 sets of 10 breaths in and 10 breaths out. Take no more than a 10 second rest between each set.

NOTES

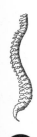

EXERCISE # 19
THE HUNDREDS - INTERMEDIATE

1. **PREREQUISITE:** Warm up stretches and 2 Sets of basic Hundreds comfortably.

2. **PURPOSE:** If you do not feel the abdominals on the BASIC Hundred then attempt this version. To strengthen the abdominals by moving the body's center of gravity.

3. **EXERCISE**: Same as the Basic Hundreds position (#18). Lower the legs to where you feel the back is just about to lift off the mat AND where the abdominals do not lift one millimeter (think of a Greyhound's stomach). B-Line. 10 Breaths in and 10 Breaths out.

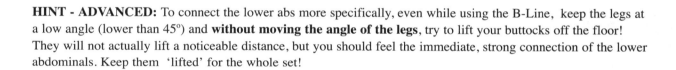

4. **KEY POINTS:** THE BACK MUST REMAIN FLAT THROUGHOUT THE EXERCISE. Keep the shoulder blades just off the floor at all times.

5. **CARE NOTES:** If the abdominals raise higher than the level of the hips and ribs, raise the legs higher and scoop the stomach. Try to B-Line more before every breath in.

6. **REPETITIONS:** Two set of 10 breaths.

HINT - ADVANCED: To connect the lower abs more specifically, even while using the B-Line, keep the legs at a low angle (lower than 45°) and **without moving the angle of the legs**, try to lift your buttocks off the floor! They will not actually lift a noticeable distance, but you should feel the immediate, strong connection of the lower abdominals. Keep them 'lifted' for the whole set!

EXERCISE # 19A
PERCUSSION BREATHING

This exercise follows the same routine as above with the following addition:
Keep the legs in parallel with the toes softly pointed. Pump the hands up and down a few centimeters, each pump being half a second. BI for 5 pumps and BO for 5 pumps until you have completed 100 pumps (or 10 breaths in and 10 breaths out).

Each pump should be as if extra air is being pumped into (or out of) the lungs. So, instead of a smooth 5 sec BI, the breathing should be 5 individual breaths in (or out) until full capacity (or deflation) is achieved.

This gives a percussion effect to the breathing and can increase the effect on the abdominals even more. Squeeze a thin pad between the knees for more abdominal effect.

CARE: If you find that the above variation is working into the neck and not very strongly in the abdominals, revert to the Basic Hundred until the abdominals are stronger.

NOTES

EXERCISE # 20
SINGLE LEG STRETCH

1. **PREREQUISITES:** Start stretches

2. **PURPOSE:** To mobilize the hip and knee joints, control abdominals, co-ordination.

3. **EXERCISE: Starting Position:**
   Lie flat on your back, both knees to the chest.

   i) Breathe Out as you contract forward, placing the right hand on the right ankle and the left hand on the right knee, elbows raised.

   ii) Extend the left leg away from the body in line with the hip and as low to the floor as possible, without the back arching. As the leg extends, turn it out and stretch through the point of the foot.

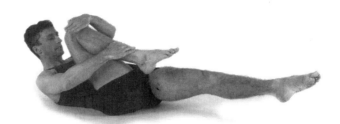

   iii) B-Line and Scoop the stomach. Breathe In as you change legs keeping the outside hand on the ankle (left hand, left ankle) and draw the left knee to the left shoulder.

4. **KEY POINTS:** Keep the shoulders relaxed, chin slightly off the chest.
   B-Line before changing legs, ribs to hips as close as possible.
   Ultimately, use the hands as a guide, do not use them to pull on the leg.
   When extending the leg, try to feel as if the inner thigh is squeezing an imaginary cushion.
   When extending the leg from the bent position, stretch through the toe along the line of the final position of the leg (do not extend into the air and then lower the leg to the ground).
   Keep the shoulders square at all times by pressing both elbows towards the hips.

5. **CARE:** If the neck starts to strain, place a cushion under the head and shoulders.

6. **REPETITIONS:** One set of ten repetitions alternating legs.

   VARIATIONS:
   1. Instead of holding on with the hands, place the wrists over the knee and ankle, with the fingers extended to the far walls. This action will ease the knee closer to the shoulder and reduce any excessive neck and shoulder work.

   2. After 6 reps extend the arms past the hips and continue to change the legs. Try to draw the knees back as close to the shoulders as before on their own! Repeat for 10 reps. Feel the abdominals!

NOTES

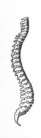

EXERCISE # 21
DOUBLE LEG STRETCH - BASIC

This exercise may appear confusing with the amount of instruction. Please persevere, it will be worth it!

1. **PREREQUISITE:** Preparation (#17), Hundreds (#18).

2. **PURPOSE:** To strengthen abdominals while moving the body's centre of gravity. To mobilize the shoulder joints. To co-ordinate breathing and arm and leg movement with abdominal control.

3. **EXERCISE: Start Position:**
   Lie on your back on the floor, knees comfortably bent to chest, slightly apart, toes pointed and touching, hands on the ankles (or shins, whichever does not hunch the shoulders), draw the ankles to the buttocks. Head on a cushion if required (Figure i).

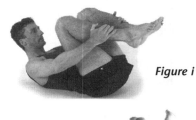
Figure i

   i) B-Line and Breathe Out as you contract forward. Extend the arms forward through the fingertips, 15cm off the floor. On the same breath out, extend the legs into the air (flexed and turned out) as low to the floor as is comfortable. Keep the back flat and scoop the stomach. Press through the heels, squeeze the inner thighs (Figure ii).

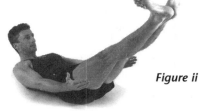
Figure ii

   ii) Breathe in as you reach through the fingers and extend the arms to a vertical position to the ceiling (don't hunch the shoulders). Hold the position for one second and B-Line harder (Figure iii).

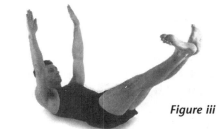
Figure iii

   iii) Keeping the B-Line, Breathe Out as you extend the arms behind the head (scraping the ears) in a big circle around and back to their start position by the hips and draw the ribs to the hips even tighter (Figure iv).

   iv) Breathe In as you return to your start position. Rest for only 1/2 a second before repeating the movement.

4. **KEY POINTS:** As the arms move from the vertical position to behind the head, ensure that the ribs stay towards the hips. This movement is always a Breath Out, depressing the rib cage.

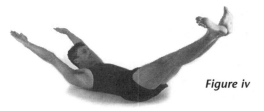
Figure iv

   Press through the heels as far as you can.
   Externally rotate the legs as much as possible.

   Stretch through the tips of the fingers at all times, do not hunch the shoulders.
   Do not allow the shoulder blades to lower to the floor on the arm circle.

5. **CARE:** If the neck feels any pressure, keep the head on a high cushion at all times.
   If the back begins to arch after several movements, raise the legs to a higher position where the small of the back stays flat on the floor. DEEP, long sigh out as the arms move (float) behind the head.

6. **REPETITIONS:** ONE SET OF 10

BREATHING SUMMARY:
   As you contract forward, raising the legs into the air:
   BI as you raise the arms from 15cm off the floor to the vertical position
   BO as you take the arms behind the head and complete the circle to the hips
   BI as you return to the rest position.

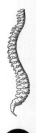

EXERCISE # 22
SINGLE LEG CIRCLES - I

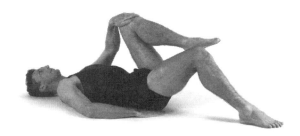

1. PREREQUISITES: Start stretches

2. PURPOSE: To isolates the adductor muscle and to mobilize the hip joint.

3. EXERCISE: Start Position:
Lie on the floor with both knees bent, thighs at 45°.
Place the hands on the floor, palms down, elbows slightly
bent and thumb and index fingers just touching the buttock
on each side. **B-Line**.
Raise the right leg to the ceiling, pointed foot and turn out the leg.
Press the right buttock into the mat and press the fingers of the right hand against the right adductor
muscle close to the groin to 'connect' the muscle.

i) Making an anti-clockwise circle, Breathe Out as you lower the leg, allowing the abdominals to lengthen.
Extend through the toes as if you were drawing a circle on the ceiling with them.
Keep the hip pressed into the mat (the circle is actually a 'D' shape with a straight line up the middle to start).

ii) Breathe In as you raise the leg to the vertical position, B-Lining.

4. KEY POINTS: Do not allow the buttock of the resting leg to lift off the fingers at all.
Keep them just touching.
FEEL the inner thigh (adductor) muscle making the circle by pressing against the fingers to establish the
connection (eventually remove the fingers).
Keep the circle high and small to start.

5. CARE: Do not push the supporting leg into the ground. This will place pressure into the lower back, raise
the buttock and can place the pelvis out of alignment.

6. REPETITIONS: Six circles in one direction, change legs. Repeat the circle in the other direction.

EASIER VARIATION - HAND ON THE KNEE

If the above is too difficult to perform for more than
4 repetitions, then try the following.
Instead of a straight leg to the ceiling, bend the knee
and place the hand on the knee.
Make a circle only as far as the hand will allow, away
from the body.
Imagine you are stirring a pot with the thigh bone.
Gradually extend the leg into the air keeping the hand
on the knee until almost fully extended.

NOTES

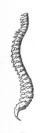

The Complete Guide to the Pilates Method

EXERCISE # 23
SIDE TO SIDE

1. **PREREQUISITES:** No major back problems, warm up stretches

2. **PURPOSE:** To strengthen the obliques while in an elongated position. To provide abdominal support for the back while in rotation.

3. **EXERCISE: Start Position:**
   Lie on your back with the knees drawn to the chest
   so they are above the lower ribs.
   Squeeze a thin pad between the knees.
   Calves parallel to the floor, feet pointed.
   Arms are placed by your sides with the palms up.

   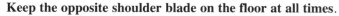

   i) Over to the side: B-Line and **Breath Out** as you
   take both knees over to the right side, but only half
   way to the floor.
   Keep the opposite shoulder blade on the floor at all times.
   Start by peeling the right hip of the floor, keeping the knees level with each other and in line with the ribs.

   ii) Return to centre: Do not press your right arm on the floor to assist the body to return to the centre.
   First **B-Line** more and then **Breathe In** as you slowly ROLL the left rib cage to the floor, imprinting the spine onto the floor from the shoulder blade to the hip.
   As you begin to roll the spine to the floor keep the knees in line with the ribs.

   THIS EXERCISE SHOULD BE FELT IN THE ABDOMINALS ONLY, NEVER IN THE BACK.

   Without stopping, Breathe Out as you flow the movement to the left side.

4. **KEY POINTS:**
   Press the knees together.
   Keep the feet parallel to the floor at all times.
   Keep the shoulders relaxed on the floor. Try not to move them.
   When comfortable (stable) with the movement, turn the head in the opposite direction to the knees to rotate throughout the length of the spine.

5. **CARE:** When taking the knees over to the side make sure they do not 'twist' at the hips.
   Both knees must move together so the lower back does not twist.
   On returning to the centre, if the hip is pulled over first, the back will tend to do the work, defeating the purpose of the exercise.

6. **REPETITIONS:** One set of ten repetitions each side.

NOTES

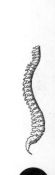

EXERCISE # 24
STOMACH STRETCH

1. **PREREQUISITE:** Hundreds (basic)

2. **PURPOSE:** Strengthen abdominals in elongation, basic strengthening of the back.

3. **EXERCISE: Start Position:**
   Lie on your stomach (prone) on the floor with your arms stretched above the head, legs extended hip distance apart, toes pointed. Forehead rested on the ground or on a cushion to keep the neck in line with the upper back.

   i) B-Line and slightly tighten your buttocks. **Breathe Out** as you extend the left arm 5cm off the ground. Imagine someone is holding your wrist and lengthening the limb out of the socket, without hunching the level line of the shoulders.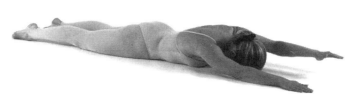

   ii) Breathe In as you keep the lengthened feeling and return to lightly touch the floor, scooping the abdominals even more.

   iii) Breathe Out as you extend the other arm.

4. **KEY POINTS:** Keep the B-Line so a ruler can easily slide between the mat and the stomach at all times Elongate the back of the neck, keep the shoulderblades pressed to the hips.

5. **CARE:** If the abdominals feel as if they are resting on the floor, the back muscles will start to do the work. Keep them supported by the abdominal contraction.
   If the back does begin to take over - stop. Attempt one more stretch each day with an increase in abdominal work.

6. **REPETITIONS:**
   One set of 10 alternating lifts

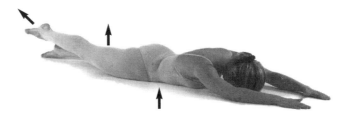

BASIC/INTERMEDIATE VARIATION
ALTERNATE LEG LIFTS

Follow the same proceedure as above, though this time use the legs instead of the arms

NOTES

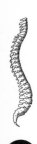

EXERCISE # 25
THE PERFECT ABDOMINAL CURL (PAC)

1. **PREREQUISITE:** Start stretches.

2. **PURPOSE:** To provide basic abdominal strength for all exercises.

3. **EXERCISE: Start Position:**
   Lie on your back on the floor, knees together,
   bent at 45° so the feet are approximately
   50-60cms from the buttocks.
   The entire back must be flat.
   Place your hands where they are most
   comfortable, either:
   a) behind the head so they are on the opposite
   shoulders to support the neck
   b) fingers interlocked behind the head with elbows wide open (photo)
   c) arms crossed on the chest.

   i) B-Line and, Breathing Out, draw the ribs as close as possible to the hips in the same horizontal plane
   as the floor until the shoulderblades come off the ground.
   Scoop the abdominals (imagine a greyhound's stomach!).

   ii) Breathe In and slowly release the abdominals 10% or to allow the torso to lower to where the
   shoulder blades almost touch the floor.

   Without stopping, repeat 10 times.

4. **KEY POINTS:** If the hands are behind the head, keep the elbows wide open. The arms are there to
   support the head, not to pull it forward. Keep the chin off the chest and the eyes focussed just above the
   knees. Imagine using the section between the ribs and the hips as a bellows. Close them on the Breath Out,
   release them on the Breath In.

5. **CARE:** Contract forward (draw the ribs to the hips) without the ribs lifting above the level of the hips
   as this may bunch the abdominals out.
   Concentrating on drawing the ribs to the hips should ease some strain on the neck.
   It is this movement which connects the abdominals, not the lift of the head, neck and shoulders.
   If the neck strains - stop.
   Move smoothly, without momentum or any jerky movements.
   If the back is arched, place the feet on a chair with the knees above the navel.

6. **REPETITIONS:** UP TO 3 SETS OF 10-12 REPS

VARIATIONS - FOR GREATER ABDOMINAL CONNECTION

1. Flex the feet so you are lightly balancing on the heels
2. Place the legs over high cushions so when they are
relaxed, the thighs do not flop open and the heels
do not touch the ground. This position greatly
reduces the connection of the front of the thighs
(quadriceps) and the inner thighs (adductors).
Keep the thighs relaxed during the entire set.
This works the abdominals more specifically with less
strain on the lower back!

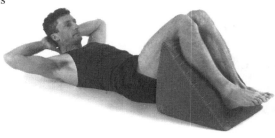

The Complete Guide to the Pilates Method

EXERCISE # 26 - I
ANKLE WEIGHTS - OUTER THIGH (ABDUCTOR)

1. **PREREQUISITES:** Nil

2. **PURPOSE:** To strengthen and tone the hip by working the outer and back of the thighs.

This exercise may be done:
a) without ankle weights (the weight of the leg may be sufficient to begin)
b) a 1 kilo weight on each leg
c) a 2 kilo weight on each leg
(advanced and men only)
For all routines lying on the side, lie with the back against a wall to ensure correct spinal posture.
Do not lean against the wall, only use it as a guide to maintain a straight back.

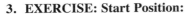

3. **EXERCISE: Start Position:**
Lie on the right side with the body in a straight line. Place the right arm under the head, extended in a line with the body, with the palm upwards.
Bend the right leg up to 45deg with the foot remaining in line with the body.
Bring the straight, left leg 15cms forward to keep the back 'flat'.
Flex the left foot and raise the leg off the ground 15cms.

The following point is important for the perfect execution of the exercise:
i) Press the left hip away from the left rib with the left hand so that the left hip sits on top of the right hip. The hips are now aligned vertically.
B-Line. Imagine the weight is on the outside of the thigh about 15cms from the hip joint.

ii) Breathe Out and lengthening through the heel, raise the leg approximately 15-30cms maximum above the height of the hip. You should feel the outer thigh of the leg working strongly.

iii) Breathing In, lower the leg to just below hip level before repeating.
Do not lower to rest the leg on the floor.

4. **KEY POINTS: Keep the hips aligned.** If the top hip continuously moves into the waist with the movement of the leg, the exercise becomes less effective.

5. **CARE: B-Line.**
If the back tends to arch, tuck the pelvis so the back is touching, but not pressing, against the wall.
As the repetitions increase, focus on lengthening through the heel.
Do not hunch the top shoulder or rotate it forward while pressing the top hip away from the rib cage.
(An alternative to pressing the top hip away is to place the left hand, palm up between the right waist and the floor, closer to the hip. Now create a gap between the palm of the hand and the waist, WITHOUT HUNCHING THE SHOULDER. As the leg lifts, attempt to INCREASE the size of this gap. If the waist touches the hand everytime the leg is raised, the leg is being raised too high causing the hip to move).

6. **REPETITIONS**: 10-20 on each leg.

ADVANCED: Bend the knee so that it is 'unlocked' for all reps.

NOTES

EXERCISE # 26 - II
ANKLE WEIGHTS - INNER THIGH (ADDUCTOR)

1. **PREREQUISITES:** Nil

2. **PURPOSE:** To strengthen, while lengthening, the inner thigh.

3. **EXERCISE: Start Position:**
   Lie on you right side and place a high cushion by the hip
   against the abdomen.
   Bend the left leg and rest it on top of the cushion.
   Right arm extended under the head,
   left hand relaxed on the floor
   Draw the right leg forward so the foot is
   30cms away from the wall behind you.
   Keep the right leg parallel and straight with the foot pointed.
   If you don't have a cushion, place the leg as in the photo.

   i) Imagine the weight is sitting high on the inner right thigh between the knee and the groin.
   B-Line and **Breathing Out**, raise the right inner thigh as high as possible without moving any other
   part of the body.

   ii) Still lengthening through the toe, **Breath In** as the leg is lowered and lightly touches the floor
   before repeating the lift. Do not rest between reps.

4. **KEY POINTS:** Do not place any pressure on the cushion to lift the lower leg.
   B-Line on the lifting and lowering of the leg.

5. **CARE: Keep the bottom leg forward of the body.**
   If the leg straightens in line with the body, the back will tend to arch and lessen the work of the
   abdominals and the inner thigh.
   If the bottom hip is uncomfortable, lie on a flat cushion.

6. **REPETITIONS:** 1 Set, 10-20 Reps.

ADVANCED:

   1. Unlock the knee and continue to lengthen through the foot and/or
   2. Turnout the lower leg from the inner thigh, without moving the hips from their vertical position.

NOTES

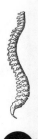

EXERCISE # 26 - III
ANKLE WEIGHT - OUTER THIGH FLEXION (ABDUCTOR)

1. **PREREQUISITES:** Ankle weights outer thigh (#26-I)

2. **PURPOSE:** To strengthen the outer thigh when the leg is at a right angle to the body.

3. **EXERCISE:** This exercise may be done:
   a) without ankle weights (the weight of the leg may be sufficient to begin)
   b) a 1 kilo weight on each leg
   c) a 2 kilo weight on each leg (advanced and men only)

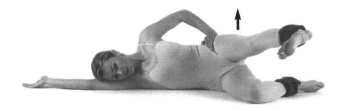

Start Position: For this exercise lie on your right side with your back against a wall to ensure correct spinal posture. **Do not lean against the wall**, only use it as a guide to maintain a straight back.
Place the right arm under the head, extended in a line with the body, with the palm facing upwards.
Bend the right leg up to 45° with the foot remaining in line with the body.
Flex the left foot and raise the leg off the ground 15cms.

i) B-Line and take the left leg as far forward as possible, at hip level, so the top knee is above the bent knee. (If the top leg can go further forward and you feel unbalanced, bend the bottom leg higher so the knees remain vertically aligned with each other.)
Breathe Out and lift the outer thigh so that the foot raises up to 15cms higher than the level of the hip. Do not lift from the foot.

ii) Breath In as the left leg lowers just below hip height.

Repeat

4. **KEY POINTS:** Attempt to keep the top hip aligned with the bottom one.
   The angle of the leg to the body will generally determine the movement in the hip joint.
   The further away from the right angle, the more stable the hip.
   Press the left hip away from the left rib with the left hand so that it sits on top of the right hip.
   The hips are now aligned vertically.

5. **CARE:** This is a difficult exercise. You may not be able to complete the same number of reps as the previous two ankle weight exercises. Do not overdo it.

6. **Repetitions:** 10-20 each side.

ADVANCED:

   1. Unlock the top knee.
   2. Turn in the leg to the floor from the thigh without moving the hip.

NOTES

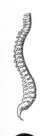

EXERCISE # 27
BACK OF THE THIGH - (HAMSTRING/BUTTOCKS)

1. **PREREQUISITE:** Ankle Weights (#26 series)

2. **PURPOSE:** To strengthen the hamstring and tone and tighten the buttocks.

3. **EXERCISE: Start Position:**
   Lie prone (on the stomach) with a flat
   cushion under the abdominals (between
   the ribs and the hips), with the forehead
   rested on the hands.
   Legs extended, turned out with feet flexed.
   Place a thick pad in the groin.

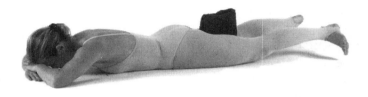

   i) B-Line and Breathe Out as you raise the legs 5cms and squeeze the pad.
   Try to touch your knees together.
   Keep the abdominals drawn up away from the cushion.
   Do not allow the hips to lift off the floor.

   ii) Breathe In and release 10% before repeating.

4. **KEY POINTS:**
   Keep the B-Line to support the lower back.
   Do not hunch the shoulders or put pressure on the elbows.

5. **CARE:** Do not raise the legs higher than 5cms to avoid the back arching.
   If the knees do touch, place a thicker pad in the groin.

6. **REPETITIONS:** 2 Sets, 10-20 Reps.

NOTES

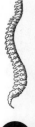

EXERCISE # 28
ARM WEIGHTS - ALL SUPINE ROUTINES

1. **PREREQUISITES:** Nil.

2. **PURPOSE:** To strengthen and mobilize the arms, chest, back and neck.
   Depending on the strength of the person, the use of weights and the amount of weight is variable.
   Heavier weights can be used for Exercise # 28-1 (openings) as no rotation of the joint is involved.
   If at home, cans of beans will do in place of weights.

3. **EXERCISE: Position for all arm weights lying on the back (supine).**

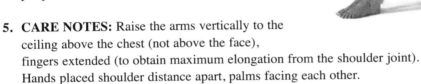

4. **KEY POINTS:** Lie on the floor or on a narrow bench, knees bent at 45°.
   B-Line. Do not allow the back to arch at any time. However, do not excessively tilt the pelvis or put pressure on the feet to force the back down.

5. **CARE NOTES:** Raise the arms vertically to the ceiling above the chest (not above the face),
   fingers extended (to obtain maximum elongation from the shoulder joint).
   Hands placed shoulder distance apart, palms facing each other.

   Do not round the shoulders off the floor or hunch the shoulders to the ears.

   'Unlock' the elbows, but continue to elongate through the length of the arm and out of the extended fingers.

   Keep the neck long and the shoulder blades always pressed towards the hips. If the neck is arched, or if there is a large gap between the back of the neck and the bench, place a cushion under the head for more comfort.

   For all the arm weight exercises, it is essential to imagine the weight is near the top of the arm, about 15cms from the shoulder. The weight becomes easier to lift in this manner and the upper arm muscles are more easily connected.

   Breathe into the chest and, on the breath out, flatten the ribs to the hips. By pressing the ribs to the hips, this has the dual benefit of connecting the upper abdominals as well as stabilizing the mid/upper back. (Imagine a slab of concrete is pressing on your chest on the breath out).

   If lying on a bench, do not allow the arms to drop below the level of the bench. If lying on the floor, do not let the weights or arms rest on the floor at any time.

   If any 'clicking' or strain occurs in the shoulder joints, reduce the range of the movement.

B-LINE AT ALL TIMES

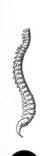

EXERCISE # 28 - 1
OPENING ARMS

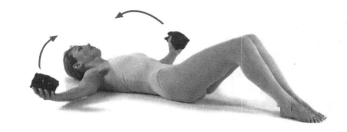

3. EXERCISE:

i) Imagine a huge beach ball is being
pumped up between your arms and
Breathing In, resist as the arms are being
pressed open to the sides.

ii) Breathing Out on the upward movement, squeeze the air out of the beach ball. Feel the chest muscles
(pectoral muscles) doing the work to raise the arms to the ceiling (imagine a pencil on your breastbone
and try to squeeze it with your chest muscles). Alternatively, get a friend to gently press against the
pectoral muscles as you press against their fingers when closing.

6. REPETITIONS: One set of up to 20 reps.

EXERCISE # 28 - 2
ALTERNATING

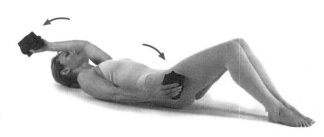

3. EXERCISE:

i) Breathing Out, extend the right arm down
to your right foot and at the same time extend
the left arm to your left ear and to a point above
your head, flattening the rib cage.

Do not hunch the left shoulder. Keep a gap between the left arm and the left ear.
Do not rest the weight above the head.
Slowly release the left chest muscle if the left arm does not extend towards the level of the ear without
the rib cage lifting.

ii) Before returning to the upright position, **B-Line** more, flatten the rib cage and, **Breathing In**,
lengthening the arms to the ceiling (the left arm by engaging the muscles in the back of the upper arm
(the triceps)). To connect this muscle and avoid shoulder strain, imaging squashing an orange under the
armpit or get a friend to gently apply pressure half way between the elbow and the shoulder and press
against this.

If the left shoulder is raised slightly towards the ear, press it towards the hip before raising the arm to the
ceiling. A better connection both above and below the shoulder joint should occur (the latissimus dorsi
will connect).

Lengthen both arms to the start position and, without stopping in the vertical position, alternate
the movement.

6. REPETITIONS: One set, 10 each side alternating.

NOTES

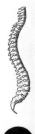

EXERCISE # 28 - 3
DOUBLE OVERHEAD ARMS

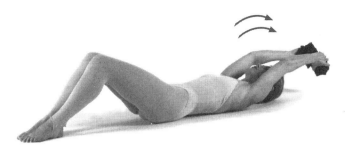

3. EXERCISE: Starting Position:
Lightly touch the fingertips (or knuckles) of
each hand together above the chest with the
elbows slightly bend outwards.

i) B-Line and **Breathing out**, extend both arms above the head to a point where, the ribs do not lift, the
back does not arch and the shoulders do not hunch.

ii) Do not rest the arms. Flatten the ribs to the hips, press the shoulder blades to the hips.

iii) Breathe In as the arms float back up to the ceiling. Imagine squashing oranges under the armpits to
connect the upper back of the arms and the latissimum dorsi.

Repeat without stopping.

6. REPETITIONS: One set of ten.

EXERCISE # 28 - 4
ARM CIRCLES

3. EXERCISE:

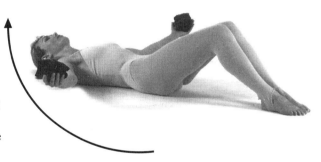

i) B-Line, Breathing In, extend both hands down
towards the heels, palms facing each other.
Do not allow the arms to go below bench level.

ii) Turn the palms up to the ceiling and **Breathing
Out** extend the arms out to the sides just above
bench or floor level until they reach as close to the
ears as is comfortable.

iii) At this point, keep moving, palms facing inwards, and **Breathe In** as the arms extend to the ceiling and
continue down to the feet. If the shoulder joints are tight the circle may be made smaller.

Remember to squeeze the imaginary oranges under the armpits to raise the arms from above the head
to the ceiling and to the feet. Try not to bend the elbows any further than the 'unlocked' position for the
entire routine.

6. REPETITIONS:
One set of ten in one direction.
One set of ten in the other direction.
Always start the circles with the movement to the heels first (inward circle).

NOTES

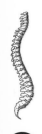

The Complete Guide to the Pilates Method

EXERCISE # 29 - 1
ARM SWINGS - ALTERNATING

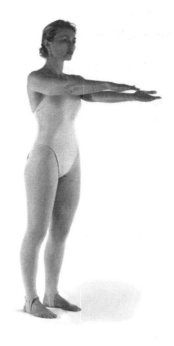

1. **PREREQUISITES:** Nil

2. **PURPOSE:** To mobilize the shoulder joints, stretch and open the
   chest (pectorals), improve thoracic and cervical posture.

3. **EXERCISE: Starting Position:**
   Stand upright on the tripods of the feet, sideways to a mirror, feet
   placed hip distance apart.

   i) B-line and raise the arms up to shoulder level with the right palm
   down and the left palm up. Lengthen through the fingertips.

   ii) Breathe Out as you take the right arm to the ceiling and the left arm
   to the floor so both palms are facing forward. Do not hunch the right
   shoulder, lengthen through the crown of the head. Flatten the ribs
   to an imaginary wall behind you on the breath out.
   This will stabilize the thoracic area and help stretch the chest muscles.

   iii) Continue to take the arms past the (vertical) line of the body.
   Look in the mirror to ensure that the back is not arching. Imagine you
   are standing against a wall and the gap between the wall and the lower
   back cannot increase. **B-Line** as firmly as possible.

   iv) Breathe In as the arms lengthen forward to the shoulder level
   position, rotate the arms and hands so the right palm is now up and
   the left palm is down and continue moving the arms, right arm to the
   floor and left arm to the ceiling.

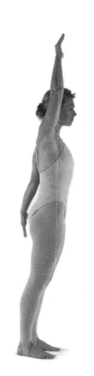

4. **KEY POINTS:** Keep the Tripods and the B-Line.
   Keep the ribs as flat as possible to the hips to prevent them
   from protruding forward and, therefore, arching the back.
   Lengthen through the fingertips.

5. **CARE:**
   Keep the neck long and upright, so it does not crane forward
   as the arms stretch past the vertical line.
   Do not hunch the shoulders.

6. **REPETITIONS:** One set, 10 reps each side alternating.

NOTES

EXERCISE # 29 - 2
ARM SWINGS - CHEST EXPANSION

1 & 2. Same as Exercise # 29 - 1.

3. **EXERCISE: Starting Position:**
   The extended arms start at navel level with the palms up to the ceiling.

   i) Breathe Out as the arms open up at a 45° angle and back behind the head at head level.
   Feel the stretch across the chest.

   ii) Breathe In as the arms return to the start position.

4. **KEY POINTS:** as in Exercise #29 - 1.

5. **CARE NOTES:**
   As the arms raise to the ceiling, press the shoulderblades to the floor.
   Do not jut the chin out.

6. **REPETITIONS:**
   One set of ten reps.

NOTES

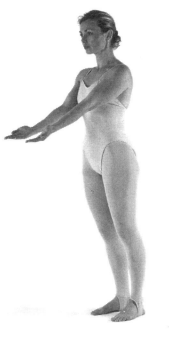

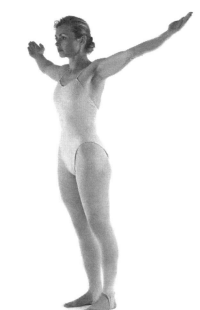

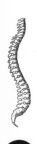

The Complete Guide to the Pilates Method

EXERCISE # 30
THE POLE

1. **PREREQUISITES:** Exercises # 28 - 1 & 2

2. **PURPOSE:** To open the chest fully and stretch the
   pectoral muscles and improve rotation of the shoulder joints.

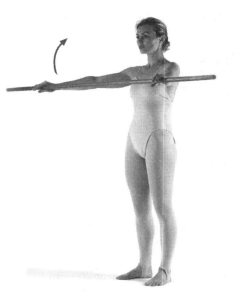

3. **EXERCISE: Starting Position:**
   Facing the mirror, B-Line and hold onto a pole / broomstick
   / IsoToner at shoulder level, hands comfortably wide apart.
   Hold the pole with only the thumb and forefinger wrapped
   around it. The other fingers remain extended. This is to
   prevent torsion in the wrist joint and straining of the neck
   once the movement has started.

   i) Lengthening the pole in front of you as if your shoulders
   were the radius of a circle, **Breathe In** and raise the pole
   to the ceiling without hunching the shoulders.

   ii) Breathe Out as the pole lengthens behind the shoulders
   and down to the floor.
   Do not bend the elbows. If they, or the shoulders/chest,
   are too tight, widen the hold on the pole.
   Lengthen the neck to the ceiling. Do not jut the chin forward.

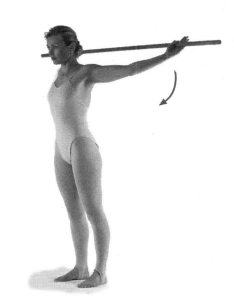

   iii) Hold the position with the pole behind your buttocks
   for the **Breath In**.
   B-Line and Breathe Out as you, once again, press the pole
   behind the shoulders to the far wall, up to the ceiling and
   forward to shoulder level.

4. **KEY POINTS:** Look in the mirror to ensure that the pole
   is always parallel to the floor.
   Keep the Tripods at all times - do not rock onto the toes
   or into the heels at any time.

5. **CARE:**
   Do not crane the neck forward.
   Do not hold the breath.
   Press the shoulders to the hips at all times.

6 **REPETITIONS:** 10 reps (backwards and forwards is one rep).

NOTES

INTERMEDIATE ROUTINE

EXERCISE # 31
HUNDREDS - ALTERNATING LEGS

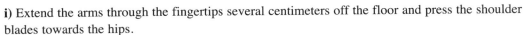

1. **PREREQUISITE:** Hundreds (#18)

2. **PURPOSE:** To work 'either side'
   of the abdominals 'separately'.

3. **EXERCISE: Starting Position:**
   Lie on your back with the legs drawn to the
   chest and holding on to the ankles, head rested
   on the floor; neck long. Contract forward (head and
   and shoulders forward, eyes on the knees, ribs drawn to the hips).
   Extend the legs vertically into the air, feet pointed, legs turned out.

   i) Extend the arms through the fingertips several centimeters off the floor and press the shoulder
   blades towards the hips.
   B-Line and **Breathe Out** as you flex the foot and lower the right leg down as far to the floor as you
   can without arching the back, the left leg remains in the air drawing slightly closer to the chest.

   ii) B-Line more and **Breathe In** as you point the right foot and raise the leg back to the vertical position.
   Change legs.

4. **KEY POINTS :**
   As the leg lowers, draw the ribs to the hips even closer to counteract any drop of the shoulders.
   Keep the shoulderblades raised off the floor when raising the leg back to vertical.
   Ensure that the vertical leg is totally straight, turned out and foot pointed.

5. **CARE:** Do not lower the leg too low if the back lifts the slightest amount.
   Lengthen the abdominals and allow the thigh muscles to 'stretch' to achieve a controlled lowering of
   the leg - imagine the hip joint is opening like a hinge.

6. **REPETITIONS:** 5-10 Reps for each leg.

NOTES

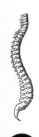

The Complete Guide to the Pilates Method

EXERCISE # 32
CO-ORDINATION

1. **PREREQUISITES:** Hundreds (#18).

2. **PURPOSE:** Co-ordination of arms, legs and breathing.
   To work the adductors, shoulders, upper back and abdominals.

3. **EXERCISE: Starting Position:**
   Lie on your back, knees comfortably to your
   chest, tailbone on the mat; hands on the knees
   with the elbows bent.

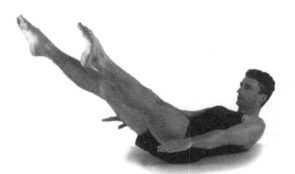

   i) B-Line and **Breathe Out** as you contract forward,
   extending the arms through the fingertips and legs
   forward as low as you can without the back arching
   (legs parallel, with toes softly pointed).

   ii) Hold the breath as you rapidly open and close the
   legs (once) just wider than shoulder distance attempting
   to connect the inner thighs for this movement.

   iii) Breathe In as you return to the start position for 1/2 a second before repeating.

4. **KEY POINTS:** Stretch through the toes as far as you can, even when opening and closing the legs.
   When returning to the rest position, draw the knees to the chest (rather than dropping the feet to the bottom).
   Keep the B-Line even when returning to the rest position.
   Do not allow them to rest until all repetitions are completed.
   Squeeze the inner thighs until the final repetition is complete.

5. **CARE:** Complete only the number of repetitions required to feel the abdominals working, where no strain
   is felt in any other part of the body.
   Focus mentally on every movement of the arms, head, neck, shoulders, legs, inner thighs and the breathing.
   Try to feel every fibre of muscle working on the contraction forward as well as the return to rest position.

6. **REPETITIONS:** One set of 10.

NOTES

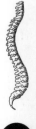

EXERCISE # 33
THE ROLL UP

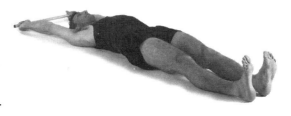

1. **PREREQUISITE:** Start Stretches, the abdominal curls (#25).

2. **PURPOSE:** Strengthen the abdominals, stretch the back.

3. **EXERCISE: Starting Position:**
   Hold onto a short pole (a small towel stretched between your hands will do). Lie on your back on a mat, arms above your head on the floor, elbows extended, legs straight, pressing through your heels.

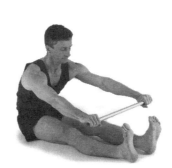

   i) B-Line and take a long **Breath In** as you raise the arms to the ceiling and bring them down to your thighs, flatten the ribs to the floor and start to roll the chin to the chest.

   ii) Breathe Out and draw the rib cage to the hips and continue rolling the head and shoulders off the floor in a smooth movement. Continue to roll each vertebra off the mat, at the same time **pressing your back into the mat** as you **peel your spine off the floor**.

   iii) Reach forward as far as you can, lengthening your chest towards your knees and the crown of your head to your toes. Hold this position and take a deep **breath into your back**.

   iv) Still reaching the arms towards the feet and pressing through the heels, **Breathe Out** as you roll back. Start by sinking into the hips and **imprinting the spine** back on the mat until the arms are above the head on the floor.
   Maintain your B-Line at all times.

4. **KEY POINTS:** Take 75% of your breath out in the first 25% of the movement or where the head and shoulders lift off the floor.
   On the return movement, take 75% of the breath out in the first 25% of the movement after sinking into the hips.
   If the lungs are too full of air, the back may not roll, but move as a stiff block.
   Correct abdominal contraction can be more easily obtained if the lungs are emptying themselves during the roll of the body.
   Keep reaching forward through the pole on the way up as if someone were pulling the pole forward for you.
   On the way down still lean forward as if someone were pulling you to your toes as you rolled down.
   This has the effect of opening up your back.

5. **CARE BEGINNERS:** If the spine is not rolling smoothly all the way (up or down) bend the knees, planting the heels into the ground and roll through the hips continually on the roll down. Keep B-Lining.

   If, on the roll up, the torso lifts rather than rolls, bend the knees more or place light weights on your feet. Engage the thighs (hip flexors) BEFORE you roll up as this will diminish the 'lifting' effect.

6. **REPETITIONS:** one set of 10.

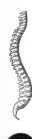

7. **BREATHING SUMMARY:**
   BO on the roll up.
   BI on the stretch forward.
   BO on the roll down.

The Complete Guide to the Pilates Method

THE PSOAS AND ITS EFFECT ON THE BACK

THE PSOAS AND ITS EFFECT ON THE BACK DURING ROLL-UPS OR CONVENTIONAL SIT-UPS IS GREATLY UNDERESTIMATED:

When resting in between each repetition (even for a fraction of a second), the torso will then lift off the floor and the hip flexors will engage at the same time, 'lurching' the body up. This is more apparent when the feet are hooked under a strap as in a gym situation.

Each repetition becomes an individual movement when the head rests for a fraction of a second. The abdominals also release for a fraction of a second and on the next repetition the body 'lurches' forward again. This is because the psoas grips. It, therefore, controls the movement and lifts the lower lumbar vertebrae, slightly distending the abdominals. This, together with weak abdominals, does not depress the psoas to allow the spine to roll up. The result is a 'lift' of the back.

Instead of completing 10 'individual' movements, keep the abdominals and hip flexors 'connected' and try to perform 10 continual movements. Think of the set as one movement comprising 10 continual parts.

If the hip flexors are continuously engaged and the abdominals are strongly B-Lined (to assist in depressing the Psoas) before the roll up begins, the chances of a 'lurch' are greatly minimized. Initially, there may be some overworking of the quadriceps. However, as the abdominals retain the engram (memory) of the rolling movement, they will supersede any hip flexor strain. When the feet are in a strap to assist in the roll up, imagine that the strap is a thin thread of cotton and any mild pull of the feet will snap that thread. This will also help to 'disengage' the psoas, even partially, and engage more of the abdominals.

The feet should remain flexed at all times. When they are in a strap and the strap is around the toes, this only engages the thighs even more. Place the strap close to the ankles.

Squeezing the inner thighs may also help slightly to alleviate the hip flexor connection.

NOTES

EXERCISE # 34
THE ROLL-OVER (OR SPINE ROLL)

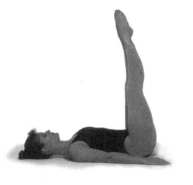

1. **PREREQUISITE:** 2 Sets of Hundreds with low legs, NO neck problems.

2. **PURPOSE:** Mobilize and massage the length of the spine and shoulders, open the vertebral spaces while flexing the spine. This exercise is similar to the yoga plough.

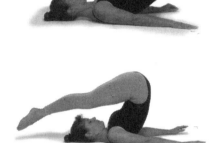

3. **EXERCISE: Starting position:**
   Lie on your back on the floor, legs vertical, feet pointed and turned out. Squeeze the back of the knees, hands by your sides, palms down. **B-Line**.

   i) Breathe Out as you draw the thighs to the rib cage (legs still straight), folding from the hips and continue rolling over smoothly. Elongating the knees to your nose until the feet touch the floor, if you can.
   Roll over <u>only</u> on to the top of the shoulders, lengthen the neck. Maintain the B-Line.

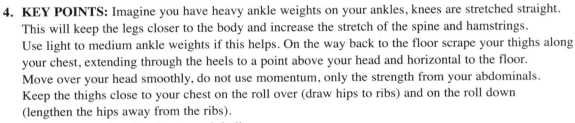

   ii) Breathe In as you turn the legs in and open them to just past shoulder width apart. Flex the feet.

   iii) Breathe Out as you roll the spine one vertebra at a time imprinting it back onto the mat until the legs are back to the start position.

4. **KEY POINTS:** Imagine you have heavy ankle weights on your ankles, knees are stretched straight. This will keep the legs closer to the body and increase the stretch of the spine and hamstrings. Use light to medium ankle weights if this helps. On the way back to the floor scrape your thighs along your chest, extending through the heels to a point above your head and horizontal to the floor. Move over your head smoothly, do not use momentum, only the strength from your abdominals. Keep the thighs close to your chest on the roll over (draw hips to ribs) and on the roll down (lengthen the hips away from the ribs). Concentrate on keeping the stomach hollow. Keep the shoulders relaxed, hardly any pressure into the arms or hands.

5. **CARE:** Do not roll onto the neck; keep the neck elongated at all times. If the feet comfortably touch the floor above the head, to obtain more stretch in the hamstrings and spine, flex the feet with legs in parallel, anchor the toes into the floor and press into the heels. Elongate the stomach on the roll down to prevent the neck arching and the shoulders lifting.

6. **REPETITIONS:** 5 reps as above and 5 reps in the reverse direction, i.e. Roll over with legs apart, feet flexed and parallel. Roll down with the legs together, turned out, feet pointed.

ADVANCED VERSION:
   Arms above the head, palms up so there is no use of the arms and more effective use of the abdominals; elbows and wrists pressed into the floor.
   On the roll down, press the elbows and shoulders into the mat; slowly release the abdominals (do not keep them contracted). Imagine they are pressing and releasing each vertebra into the mat.
   This will prevent the head and shoulders from lifting off the mat.

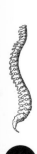

EXERCISE # 35
SINGLE LEG CIRCLES

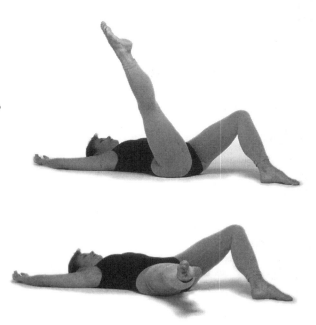

1. **PREREQUISITES:** Single leg circle I (#22).

2. **PURPOSE:** To isolates the adductor muscle and to mobilize the hip joint.

3. **EXERCISE: Starting position:**
   Lie on the floor with both legs bent.
   Place the arms extended out to the sides
   on the floor, palms up. B-Line.
   Raise the right leg to the ceiling,
   point the foot and turn out the leg.
   Press the left buttock into the mat.

   i) Making an anti-clockwise circle,
   Breathe Out as you take the leg across the body
   to the left and then lower the leg to the floor,
   allowing the abdominals to stretch.
   Extend through the toes while making a large circle out to the far right.

   ii) Breathe In as you raise the leg to the vertical position: **B-Line**.
   The circle is a rapid movement as the leg is lowered and extended to the side.
   It is a slower movement as it is raised and crosses the body.

   Eventually, attempt to make the circle as close to the floor as possible without the opposite hip moving at all.

4. **KEY POINTS:** FEEL the inner thigh (adductor) muscle making the circle.
   Keep the circle high and small to start. Do not allow the leg to lower too far if the back arches.
   Press the fingers of the right hand into the right adductor to feel the connection for this muscle.
   Keep a tripod on the left foot.

5. **CARE:** Do not push the arms onto the floor.

6. **REPETITIONS:** Six circles in one direction, change legs. Repeat the circle in the other direction.

ADVANCED: Extend the bent leg onto the floor, foot flexed.

NOTES

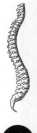

EXERCISE # 36
DOUBLE LEG STRETCH II - (LOWERING AND RAISING)

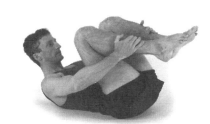

1. **PREREQUISITE:** Preparation (#17),
   Double Leg Stretch (#21), Hundred (#31), Co-Ordination (#32).

2. **PURPOSE:** Abdominal strength and control when moving the lower limbs, breathing control, shoulder mobility.

3. **EXERCISE: Starting position:**
   Complete the starting position of the basic double leg stretch (#21), this time keeping the legs just past the vertical position, away from the body. Complete the arm circle.

   i) Hold this position and take a deep **Breath In**.

   ii) Breathe Out as you lower the legs, as low as you can without lifting the back, feet flexed and turned out, squeeze the inner thighs (Figure i).

   iii) B-Line harder and **Breathe In** as you raise the legs back to the vertical position, still squeezing the inner thighs.

   iv) Breathe Out as you extend the hands to the ceiling and continue, on the same breath to complete a second circle with the arms (Figure ii).

   v) Breathe In and return to the start position (Figure iii).

   Figure i

   Figure ii

   Figure iii

4. **KEY POINTS:** When lowering the legs, press through the heels.
   Keep the shoulderblades just off the floor at all times.
   It is important not to allow the head and shoulders to lower as the legs lower.
   This may arch the back, which may then strain when lifting the legs.
   Feel as if the abdominals are flattening and lengthening to allow the legs to lower.
   When raising the legs, B-Line first and feel as if the hips are drawing to the rib cage.
   Feel as if the action of the abdominals contracting is what raises the legs into the air.

5. **CARE:** If the exercise is too challenging to start, return to the rest position after the legs have been raised - do not complete the second circle.
   If, after several repetitions, the back begins to arch, do not lower the legs too far.

6. **REPETITIONS:** One set of ten, half a second rest between each repetition.

BREATHING SUMMARY:
   Breathe Out contract forward.
   Breathe In arms to vertical.
   Breathe Out arms around in big circle.
   Breathe In hold position with hands by the sides.
   Breathe Out lower the legs.
   Breathe In raise the legs.
   Breathe Out second full circle (optional).
   Breathe In rest for 1/2 sec.

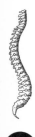

The Complete Guide to the Pilates Method

EXERCISE # 36 - VARIATIONS
VARIATIONS OF THIS VERSION TO MAKE THE ABDOMINALS WORK HARDER

1. **PREREQUISITES:** Double Leg Stretch (#38).

   Follow all the instructions as in the Double Leg Stretches and then continue as per the instructions that follow.

2. **ARMS TO CEILING:**
   After completing the first circle,
   i) Breathe In as you raise your arms to vertical, then
   ii) Breathe Out as you lower the legs and continue as before (Figure i).

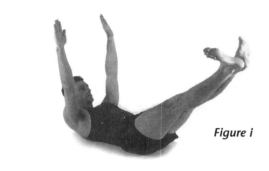

Figure i

3. **ARMS TO EARS:**
   After completing the first circle,
   i) Breathe In as you raise your arms past the vertical to the same line as your ears, then
   ii) Breathe Out as you lower the legs and continue as before (Figure ii).

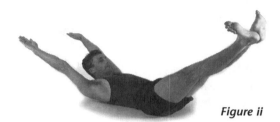

Figure ii

4. **EXPANSION:**
   After completing the first circle,
   i) Breathe In as you raise the arms vertically, then
   ii) Breathe Out as you lower the right leg and extend the right arm to the right ear,
   iii) Breathe In as the raise the leg and arm,
   iv) Breathe Out as you repeat with the other arm and leg.
   Continue as before (Figure iii).

NOTES

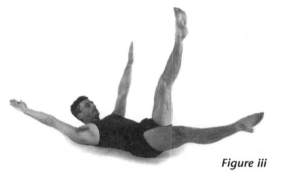

Figure iii

EXERCISE # 37
ROLLING

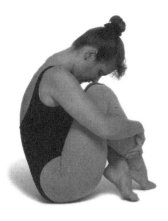

1. **PREREQUISITE:** Roll up (#33) , PACurls (#25).

2. **PURPOSE:** To stretch and mobilize the spine.

3. **EXERCISE: Starting position:**
   Sit on the floor on a mat with your heels drawn to your tailbone,
   forehead rested between the knees that are slightly apart.
   Cross your right ankle over your left, clasp the hands on the top ankle.
   Hold tight. B-Line.

   i) Sink into your hips and round your back. At the same time
   Breathe Out as you roll smoothly onto your spine up to your
   shoulderblades, keeping your heels to the tailbone, lengthen your neck.

   ii) Breathe In as you pull your hands sharply to the floor to initiate the
   movement back to the upright position. Balance on your tailbone with
   the toes lightly touching the floor.

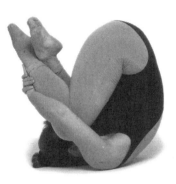

   Repeat.

4. **KEY POINTS:** Keep the heel close to the tailbone.
   Only roll onto the shoulders, not the neck.
   Sink into the hips to start the movement, this will help 'curl' the tailbone to start the smooth roll.
   You may find that you will roll to one side of the mat, this will even itself out as you perform more
   sets and gain better balance.

5. **CARE:** If the back has any 'flat spots' at all, stop. These are sections of the spine which do not roll
   smoothly; more effort is then spent on 'lifting' the body off the ground, than on rolling smoothly.

6. **REPETITIONS:** ONE SET OF 10 ROLLS.

NOTES

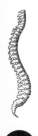

The Complete Guide to the Pilates Method

EXERCISE # 38
SINGLE LEG STRETCH WITH ROTATION (CRISS-CROSS)

1. **PREREQUISITE:** Perfect Abdominal Curl (#25), Single leg stretch (#20).

2. **PURPOSE:** To strengthen the obliques.

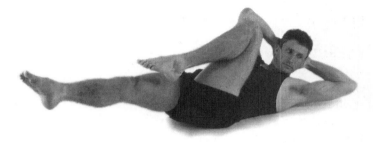

3. **EXERCISE:** In essence, this exercise is the same as the Curls and Single Leg Stretch combined.
   Starting position: Lying on the floor, contract forward with hands behind the head, elbows open.

   i) **Breathe Out** and Curl the right armpit towards the left knee, drawing the knee towards the left shoulder. The right leg is extended, pointed and turned out, as low to the floor as possible without the back lifting. Scoop the stomach.

   ii) **Breathing In**, change legs and *release* the torso until the shoulderblades almost touch the floor.

   Repeat to the other side.

4. **KEY POINTS:** Keep the shoulderblades off the floor at all times.
   Keep the elbows open.
   Turn the head and shoulders and look to the side for maximum rotation of the torso (where the eyes go, the body follows).
   Keep the hips still, planted into the mat.
   B-Line at all times.
   Be sure to extend the legs in line with the hip, not out to the sides.

5. **CARE:** Keep the elbows open so there is no strain on the neck.
   Keep the chin off the chest, eyes forward at 45° except when turning.
   When turning to the side keep both shoulders off the floor.

6. **REPETITIONS:** One set of ten to each side.

NOTES

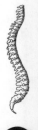

EXERCISE # 39
STOMACH STRETCH - ALTERNATING ARMS AND LEGS

1. **PREREQUISITE:** Stomach Stretches (#24).

2. **PURPOSE:** To strengthen back muscles.

3. **EXERCISE: Starting position:**
   Lie on the stomach with arms and legs
   extended shoulder width apart. Place a
   small flat cushion between the hips and
   the ribs to help support the B-Line.
   Forehead rested on the floor or on a
   cushion. Legs pointed and turned out.

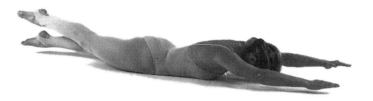

   i) B-Line and **Breathing Out**, lift and lengthen the opposite arm and leg less than 5 cms off the floor.
   Pinch the buttocks, but do not grip. At the same time imagine a greyhound's stomach in the abdominals.

   ii) Keeping the buttocks pinched, **Breathe In** as you slowly lower the arm and leg and change to the
   other arm and leg.

4. **KEY POINTS:** B-Line to prevent the back arching.
   Allow the movement to flow smoothly.
   Keep the muscles of the arm and leg, which are in contact with the floor, 'holding' (not fully rested).
   Relax the neck, drawing the shoulderblades to the hips.
   Lengthen through the tips of the fingers and toes.

5. **CARE:** If any twinges are felt in the back, draw the stomach in harder. If this is of no assistance,
   stop the exercise after only a few repetitions.
   Lengthen the neck. If the head is dropped below the level of the shoulders, place the forehead
   on a higher cushion, where the neck is not arching.

6. **REPETITIONS:** 6-10 lifts each side.

NOTES

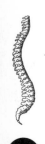

EXERCISE # 40
SINGLE LEG KICK

1. **PREREQUISITE:** Hundreds (#19) and a strong back.

2. **PURPOSE:** Firm the hamstrings and buttocks, strengthen abdominals in an elongated position, stretch the front of the thighs.

3. **EXERCISE: Starting Position:** Lie on your stomach on the floor, legs extended, toes pointed.

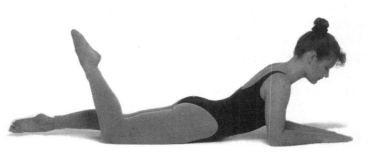

   i) B-Line and rise up onto your elbows keeping them directly below your shoulders, palms down pressed into the mat. Lengthen through the crown of the head without arching the neck. Keep the hips pressed into the mat and lift your chest as high as you can, stretching the abdominals, but keep B-Lining to support the back. Stretch through the toes, squeeze the buttocks firmly, lift the feet just off the ground.

   ii) Breathe Out as you kick the right foot to your buttock twice rapidly.
   The second kick only lowers half way to the floor and kicks to the buttock with a flexed foot.

   iii) Then point the foot and **Breathe In** as you lower the leg to the floor.

   Change legs.

4. **KEY POINTS:** If the hips lift off the floor and the back feels tight, extend the elbows further in front of you, so the back is longer.
   Make sure the hip bones stay on the floor.
   Keep the ribcage lengthened away from the hips.
   Breathe out sharply and fast for each kick.

5. **CARE:** If you feel the back starting to take any pressure, B-Line more firmly.
   If the pressure continues - stop the exercise.
   Keep the back of the neck in a long curve in line with the upper part of the back.
   Use the pressure of the palms of the hands to stabilize yourself, fingers extended.

6. **REPETITIONS:** One set of five kicks on each leg alternating.

BREATHING SUMMARY:
   Breathe Out, out on the kick, kick.
   Breathe In when lowering the leg.

NOTES

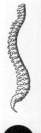

EXERCISE # 41
DOUBLE LEG KICK

1. **PREREQUISITE:** Single leg kick (#40).

2. **PURPOSE:** Firm the buttocks, hamstrings; strengthen the back, open the chest.

3. **EXERCISE: Starting position:**
   Lie on your stomach with your head turned
   to the right. Legs straight, feet pointed.
   One hand holding the other, behind your
   back as high up towards the shoulderblades
   as you can with elbows touching the floor.
   B-Line and 'zip' up the stomach (Figure i).

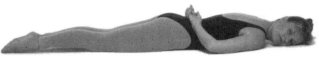

Figure i

   i) Breathe Out as you rapidly kick your feet together
   to your buttocks three times (Figure ii).

   ii) Breathe In as you then stretch the legs away as
   high as you can from the body, at the time stretch
   your hands towards your feet, still holding them
   together; and

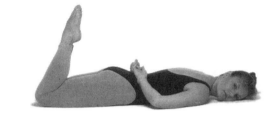

Figure ii

   iii) Lift your chest off the floor as high as
   possible without arching your neck, looking
   towards the ceiling (Figure iii).

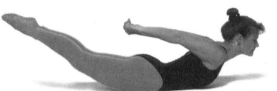

Figure iii

   iv) Breathe In as you return to the start position with
   your head turned in the other direction.

4. **KEY POINTS:** Press the shoulderblades to the hips and keep the neck long.
   As you lift the chest off the ground, flatten the ribs in a smooth line to the abdominals.
   Squeeze the buttocks firmly throughout the routine.

5. **CARE:** Reduce the intensity or lift of the movement if you feel tightness in the shoulders,
   neck or lower back.

6. **REPETITIONS:** one set of 10 kicks alternating the head each time.

BREATHING SUMMARY:
   Breathe Out as you kick 3 times.
   Breathe In as you lift and lengthen.
   Breathe Out as you lower the torso and repeat the kicks.

NOTES

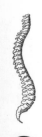

The Complete Guide to the Pilates Method

EXERCISE # 42
SWAN DIVE I (ROCKING PRESS-UP I)

1. **PREREQUISITES:** Quad Stretches (#13), Curls (#25), Stomach stretches (#39)

2. **PURPOSE:** Back strengthening, Control.

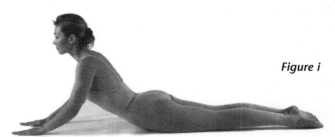

Figure i

3. **EXERCISE: Starting position:**
   Lie on the stomach in the press-up position, hands close to the shoulders, fingers forward Lengthen through your toes with your legs in a comfortable position (parallel). B-Line and keep the buttocks tight, but not gripping.

   i) Raise the legs slightly off the ground and, Breathing Out, straighten your arms rising off the mat, letting your thighs contact the mat. Lengthen the head high and back, without feeling any pressure along the spine (Figure i).

   LOCK YOUR BODY INTO THIS POSITION.

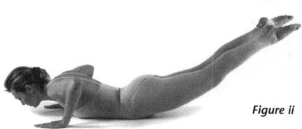

Figure ii

   ii) Breathing In, bend the arms and rock forward. The legs should raise into the air. Reaching the toes to the ceiling, roll as far forward onto your breastbone as possible (Figure ii).

   iii) Immediately rock back into the straight arm position (Figure i).

4. **KEY POINTS:** If this movement is uncomfortable in the hip area, place a cushion under the hips. Keep the movement smooth at all times with rhythmic breathing.

5. **CARE:** Keep lengthening through the crown of the head and through the point of the toes. Reverse the breathing if it is more comfortable, but keep B-Lining. Keep the shoulder blades pressed to the hips.

6. **REPETITIONS:** 3 to 8 times.

NOTES

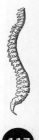

EXERCISE # 42 - I
SWAN DIVE II (ROCKING PRESS-UP II)

The movement is the same as Exercise # 42.

i) After straightening the arms, in a rapid movement lift them up off the floor in line with your ears (Figure i).

Figure i

ii) Extend your arms forward with the palms facing down and your body will rock forward.

iii) Breathing Out, rock as far forward onto your breastbone as possible before rocking back as high as you can, breathing in (Figure ii).

Figure ii

Continue rocking and keep the movement as smooth as possible.

Complete 3 - 8 repetitions.
Follow all the other instructions as Exercise # 42 (Rocking Press-up I)

EXERCISE # 43
SWIMMING

1. **PREREQUISITE:** Hundreds (#19), Stomach Stretch (#39)

2. **PURPOSE:** Strengthen back muscles, mobilize hips and shoulders.

3. **EXERCISE: Starting position:**
   Lie on the floor with the arm and legs extended, feet slightly apart.

   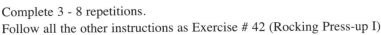

   i) B-Line, lightly tighten the buttocks and lift the arms, chest and legs 15cms off the floor. Lengthen through the tips of the fingers and toes, keeping the shoulders and pelvis square. Shoulder blades to hips.

   ii) From this start position, raise the right arm and left leg 10cms higher.
   Breathe Out as you quickly alternate the arms and legs for five beats.

   iii) Breathe In for 5 beats.

4. **KEY POINTS:** Keep the B-Line.
   Shoulders relaxed, shoulderblades to hips.
   Extend the arms and legs through the fingertips and toes.

5. **CARE:** Keep the legs to a height where the abdominals are pulled away from the floor or the back may take over.

6. **REPETITIONS:** One set of 10 breaths in and out.

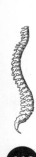

NOTES

EXERCISE # 44
SPINE ROTATION (SPINE TWIST)

1. **PREREQUISITE:** Start stretches.

2. **PURPOSE:** To provide mobility in the spine in rotation, to focus on lifting out of the hips.

3. **EXERCISE: Starting position:**
   Sit upright on your sit bones on a mat, legs straight in front of you, press through the heels and keep them together. Without hunching the shoulders, raise your arms to shoulder height, palms down, stretching through the fingertips; lift the ribs away from the hips and stretching the crown of your head to the ceiling (Figure i).

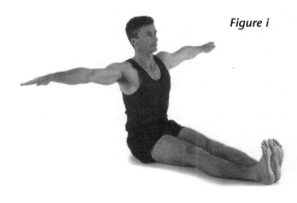

Figure i

   i) B-Line and **Breathe Out deeply** as you rotate the body to the right as far as you can. Initiate the movement from the rib cage and, flattening the ribs as you rotate, maintain the erect posture. Imagine you are turning on the base of your spine (Figure ii).

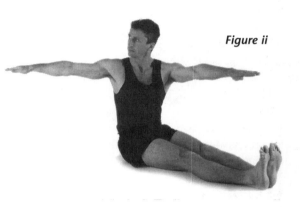

Figure ii

   ii) When you have rotated as far as you can, hold the position for half a second (keeping the ribs flat and the posture erect), **Breathe Out** more as you rotate a little further, this time turning the right shoulder blade as far back as possible.

   iii) Breathe In as you return to the start position and without stopping, smoothly flow into a rotation in the other direction.

4. **KEY POINTS:** Keep lifted out of the hips.
   Keep the shoulder blades to the hips at all times.
   Turn the head with the shoulders and feel the movement loosening the rib cage area.
   Do not allow the hips to move.

5. **CARE:** Only do the number of repetitions that are comfortable for the neck and shoulders.
   Perform the movement slowly without much rotation to start and, as you warm up, go faster increasing the rotation each time.

6. **REPETITIONS:** 10 to each side.

NOTES

EXERCISE # 45
SPINE STRETCH

1. **PREREQUISITE:** All start stretches, hamstrings and quadriceps.

2. **PURPOSE:** To stretch the spine and the hamstrings.

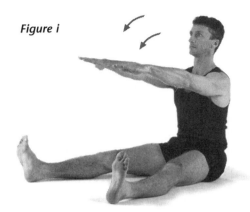

Figure i

3. **EXERCISE: Starting position:**
   Sit upright on the sit bones with the legs slightly wider than shoulder distance apart, feet flexed, knees pressed to the floor. Arms to the ceiling. Ribs lifted vertically from the hips, shoulderblades to hips.

   i) **Breathe Out** as you curl the chin down to the rib cage, then nose to B-Line.
   Extend the arms in front of you as far forward as possible without hunching the shoulders, keeping the nose towards the B-Line (Figure i).

   ii) **Breathe In** and hold the position.

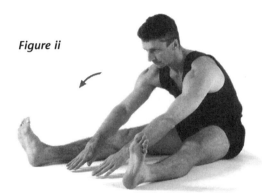

Figure ii

   iii) **Breathing Out** lengthen the spine forward as far as possible (Figure ii).

   iv) Hold the stretch, **Breathing In**.

   v) **Breathe Out** as you curl the spine back to the upright position, still reaching through the fingertips as far forward as possible.

4. **KEY POINTS:** If you feel any discomfort in the back of the knees, bend them slightly.
   Keep the shoulderblades pressed to the hips.
   Curl on the return to upright. Start by B-Lining and then stacking the vertebrae one at a time on top of each other, lifting the ribs from the hips, keeping the nose to the B-Line until the very end.
   Then life the head upright.
   Focus on deep breathing at all times.

5. **CARE:** Do not force the movement. As you complete more of these you will find you shall gradually become looser.

6. **REPETITIONS:** One set of ten stretches.

BREATHING SUMMARY:
   Breathe Out on curling the nose to the B-Line.
   Breathe In hold.
   Breathe Out stretch forward.
   Breathe In hold.
   Breathe Out return to upright.

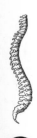

NOTES

EXERCISE # 46
OPEN LEG ROCKER

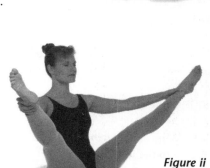

Figure i

1. **PREREQUISITE:** Start stretches, Hamstrings, Crunches, Roll-over.

2. **PURPOSE:** To improve balance.

3. **EXERCISE: Starting position:**
   Sit tall on the floor with your knees bent open, toes pointed and close
   to your tailbone, hands on the ankles inside the open knees (Figure i).

   i) B-Line and, balancing on your tailbone, straighten your legs
   into the air to form a V. Arms should be straight (Figure ii).

   ii) Curve your back into a C shape by sinking into your
   hips (with control), and
   Breathe Out as you smoothly roll along your spine to the
   top of your shoulders (Figure iii).

   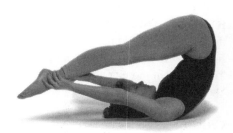

   Figure ii

   iii) Breathe In as you roll back to the upright position sitting tall,
   chin up, spine long. Repeat.

4. **KEY POINTS:** A great deal of balance and abdominal control
   is required for this exercise.
   When the legs are extended into the air, try to align the toes
   with the top of your head.
   Keep the ribs to the hips on the roll over and the roll up.
   Press the abdominals in the direction of the hips as hard
   as possible for both movements.
   On the roll up, flatten the ribs as you sit in the upright
   position as if you have a rod up your spine from the tailbone
   to the crown of your head.

Figure iii

5. **CARE:** Roll over only onto the top of the shoulders, keeping your chin to your ribcage.
   If you feel unbalanced as you roll into the upright position, bend the knees slightly to gain
   more control over the movement.
   Roll smoothly through the spine - no flat spots.

BEGINNERS HINT:
   If you unable to gain control on this movement, start with the start position and try straighten the legs open,
   then:
   Breathe Out as you close the legs together, trying to extend the lower back.
   Keeping your balance, Breathe In as you open the legs, sitting taller, flatten the ribcage.
   Breathe Out as you bend the knees back to the start position.
   Repeat 6-10 times.

6. **REPETITIONS:** One set of 6.

BREATHING SUMMARY:
   Breathe In extend the legs.
   Breathe Out roll back.
   Breathe In roll upright.

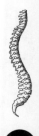

EXERCISE # 47
CORKSCREW - BASIC

1. **PREREQUISITE:** Hundreds Alternating (#31).

2. **PURPOSE:** Oblique and abdominal strength, hip and lower back mobility.

3. **EXERCISE: Starting position:**
   Lie on the floor, arm by the sides, palm down
   Extend both legs vertically into the air, feet pointed and turned out,
   squeeze the back of the knees together.

   i) B-Line and **Breathe Out** as both legs lower out to the right side
   and away from the body into a circle (photo).

   ii) Breathe In as the legs return to the vertical position.

   iii) B-Line and Breathe Out as the legs then reverse direction
   and go to the left.

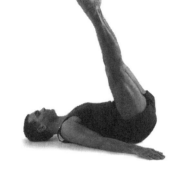

   Because of this continual change of direction, the obliques and abdominals are required to also change
   their direction of control. This constant *redirection* of the muscle provides a greater challenge than 10
   circles in the one direction.

4. **KEY POINTS:** As the legs lower away from the body, *lengthen and flatten* the abdominals to prevent
   the back from arching.
   Imagine the movement is being performed from the inner thighs near the groin.
   You will gain more control this way.
   Do not press on the arms.

5. **CARE:** Start with small corkscrews where the hips do not move off the floor then, as you gain more
   confidence and control, make the corkscrew bigger.

6. **REPETITIONS:** One set of 6 to 10 in each direction.

EXERCISE 47 - I
CORKSCREW I - INTERMEDIATE

This exercise is similar in all aspects to Corkscrew, except the circle is bigger.

EXERCISE: Make the circle bigger to work the abdominals more. As this becomes easier, take the arms out
away from the body, keeping the palms up. If the palms are down there is more tendancy to push the hands on
the floor to keep your control, rather than use the abdominals; this would also strain the neck and shoulders.
As you become more proficient with this version, keep extending the arms above shoulder height on the floor
and the circle close to the floor! (Do not allow the shoulders to lift off the floor). This is abdominal control
at its best.

NOTES

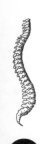

EXERCISE # 47 - II
CORKSCREW II - ADVANCED

1. **PREREQUISITE:** Corkscrew (#47-I), roll-over (#34).

2. **PURPOSE:** Strengthen the abdominals, obliques, spine; mobilize the spine and hips.

3. **EXERCISE: Starting position:** Lie flat on your back on the floor; legs vertical, turned out, feet pointed, squeeze the back of the knees; arms by you sides, palms down (Figure i).

   i) Breathe Out and Roll over onto the shoulders to the roll over position (Exercise # 33) (Figure ii).

   ii) Hold the position for the **Breathe In**.

   iii) Breathe Out as you take the legs to the right side of the body, rolling the hips to the left (Figure iii).
   Roll onto the right side of the body, lowering the legs away into a circle.

   iv) Breathe In as you roll back up onto the left side of the body into the roll over position.

   v) Breathe Out as your now reverse the movement, rolling onto the left side of the body.

4. **KEY POINTS:** The further over into the roll-over you are, the better.
   However, remain on the top of the shoulders only.
   The bigger the circle (out to the sides and down to the floor) the more challenging the exercise.
   Keep the movement fluid and the roll smooth.
   Try to place the least amount of pressure possible on the hands.
   Keep the shoulders relaxed, use the abdominals.
   Keep the legs turned out, stretching through the toes.
   B-Line at all times!

5. **CARE:** If the back arches too much, or the shoulders do most of the work - stop the exercise.
   Keep the breathing smooth and deep - do not hold your breath.
   Keep the back of the neck long and pressed into the mat.
   Keep the shoulder blades to the hips.

6. **REPETITIONS:** Up to 5 Complete Movements.
   (One corkscrew is a roll onto the side in each direction).

BREATHING SUMMARY:
   Breathe Out as you roll the back to the floor and stretch the legs away.
   Breathe In as you roll onto the shoulders with the legs above the head.

NOTE: It may be an idea to review the notes on breathing at this point. See General Breathing Rules.

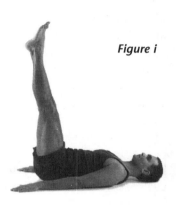
Figure i

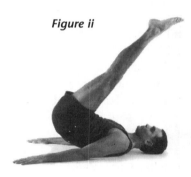
Figure ii

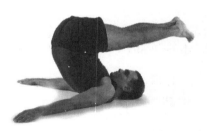
Figure iii

EXERCISE # 48
THE SAW

1. **PREREQUISITES:** Spine Stretch (#45).

2. **PURPOSE:** To provide basic rotation of the spine concentrating on the rib cage to provide this movement.

3. **EXERCISE: Starting position:** Sit upright on the floor as if there were a rod up your spine. Extend the arms out to the sides, parallel to the floor, reaching through the fingertips, as if a pole were extended from one finger tip, through the shoulders, to the other fingertip (Figure i).

   Figure i

   i) Breathe Out as you rotate to the torso to the right by turning the rib cage and at the same time reaching forward with the left hand towards the outside of the right foot (Figure ii).

   ii) Keep breathing out as you imitate a sawing action with the edge of the right hand half way up the outside edge of the foot for two short strokes. Two sharper breaths out for each of the sawing movements will help to stretch further.

   Figure ii

   iii) Breathe In as you return to the upright position by rolling the rib cage back using the oblique muscles.

   iv) Stretch to one side, return to upright; stretch to the other side with a continuous flowing movement. Return to upright.

4. **KEY POINTS:** As you reach forward to saw off the foot,
   rotate the torso as if you are trying to turn your chest towards the ceiling.
   Lengthen through the crown of the head.
   Press both buttocks firmly into the floor at all times.
   Keep the feet flexed.
   Do not rest the head on the shoulder when rotating the torso.

5. **CARE:** If you cannot reach the foot, do not force it. It is more important to control the rotation from the anterior part of the torso.
   Rotate only as far as is comfortable. Reach only as far as is comfortable. For some of you this may be only 50% of that shown in the photograph. This is perfect - gradually progress from here.

6. **REPETITIONS:** Up to ten stretches to each side continuously alternating sides.

BREATHING SUMMARY:
   Breathe Out Rotate, reach and two further short breaths out on the saw.
   Breathe In and Rotate back to the upright position.

NOTES

EXERCISE # 49
SIDE KICK I

1. **PREREQUISITES:** Start stretches, Hundreds (#31).

2. **PURPOSE:** Mobilize the hips, stretch the hamstring, strengthen the lower back.

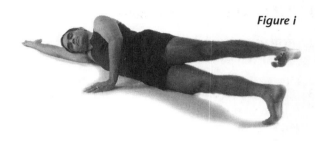
Figure i

3. **EXERCISE: Starting position**
Lie on the floor on your right side, with your head resting on your right arm, elbow in line with the body, left hand palm down on the mat by your waist, balancing on your right hip.

i) Keeping your legs straight, bring them slightly forward, both feet flexed lengthening through the heels. Right toes pressed into the floor. Lift the left leg slightly to hip level, keep the foot flexed and **B-Line** (Figure i).

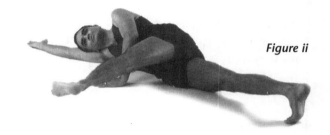
Figure ii

ii) Take a deep **Breathe In** as you kick the left leg forward as far as you can, pressing through the heel. Keep the spine straight (Figure ii).

Figure iii

iii) At the end of the kick, do a further, smaller kick inhaling an extra breath to expand the lungs more.

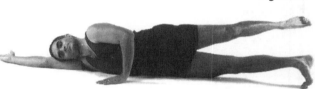

iv) Point your foot and **Breathe Out** as you kick your leg back in a sweeping motion, stretching through the top of the thigh, **B-Line harder** (Figure iii). Flatten the rib cage and keep the back as straight as you can.

v) Flex the foot and press through the heel for the next kick forward.

4. **KEY POINTS:** Stabilize your centre and, as if your hip were the centre of a circle, lengthen through the heel and toe reaching past the outer rim of the circle.
Keep the shoulders stable and chin lifted.
Lengthen through the crown of the head.
To keep the top hip directly above the bottom one, create a small gap between the waist and the floor.

5. **CARE:** If any strain is felt in the back, discontinue the exercise.
If you feel the hip bone on the mat, place a flat cushion under the hip.

6. **REPETITIONS:** 10 kicks each side.

BREATHING SUMMARY:
Breathe In kick forward, extra breath in at the stretch.
Breathe Out kick back.

EXERCISE # 50 - I
SIDE LEG LIFTS

1. **PREREQUISITES:** Hundreds (#31).

2. **PURPOSE:** To strengthen side muscles of the waist (Quadratus Lumborum), obliques and the outside of the thigh (tensor fascia lata).

3. **EXERCISE: Starting position:**
   Lie on your left side with your head resting on your left arm, elbow in line with the body. Right hand lightly placed on the floor by the waist. Keep the legs parallel, slightly in front of the body and toes pointed. There should be a small gap between the left waist band and floor. Tuck the pelvis (posteriorly) to assist in maintaining a flatter back.

   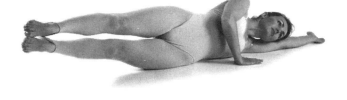

   i) B-Line and **Breathe Out** as you lift both legs as high as you can without leaning the hips backwards.

   ii) Breathe In as you lower the legs slowly until they almost touch the floor.

   Repeat.

4. **KEY POINTS:** Maintain the gap between the waistband and the floor.
   Deep Sigh on the breath out.

   For beginners, to prevent the hips rolling back, keep your back flat against a wall without leaning against it.

5. **CARE:** If there is an arch in the back, flatten this by connecting the lower abdominals more with the posterior tuck. If there is still a fair sized arch keep both legs further forward of the straight line of the body, so the back does not excessively engage.
   Keep the supporting hand relaxed. Do not use it to push on the floor as this will hunch the shoulder.
   Place a thin cushion between the thighs and squeeze as you lift, for more control and tone of the adductor muscles.
   If you find pressure on the bottom hip as you lift the legs, place a flat cushion under the hip.

6. **REPETITIONS:** 10 LIFTS THEN CHANGE AND REPEAT ON THE OTHER SIDE.

ADVANCED: Raise your left hand behind your head, with the elbow behind your ear and to the ceiling. Greater balance is required for this version.

EXERCISE # 50 - II
SIDE LEG KICK

Lie in the same **start position** as in Side Leg Lifts (#50) above.

i) Turnout the top leg so the knee cap is facing the ceiling, foot pointed.
ii) B-Line and **Breathe In** as you kick up to the ceiling. Do not lean back.
iii) Flex the foot and **Breathe Out** as you press through the heel lowering back to the other foot.
Repeart 10 times, then change sides.

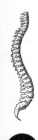

EXERCISE # 51
PELVIC CURL

1. **PREREQUISITES:** Nil.

2. **PURPOSE:** To help open and mobilize the lower back. To connect the lower abdominals. This exercise is best done with the legs on a chair.

3. **EXERCISE: Starting position:**
   Lie on your back with feet on a chair
   and hip distance apart. The angle of
   the thigh bone should be 90° to the floor.
   If the feet are too close to the buttocks,
   more pressure will be applied to the
   lower back when doing the movement.

   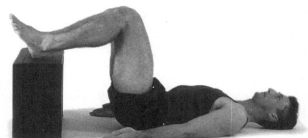

   i) With the palms facing up by your sides,
   B-Line and **Breathing Out**, draw the
   hipbones to the rib cage and continue to do
   so until the pelvis tilts off the floor about 5-10cms.

   ii) **Breathing In**, slowly release the hips down to the floor. Do not disconnect the abdominal control.

4. **KEY POINTS:** It may help to gently press the fingers of one hand into the lower abdominals to find the connection of the abdominal muscles.

5. **CARE**: Do not press on the arms or feet to achieve this movement.
   Do not tense the shoulders, lengthening the neck.
   Do not press on the heels.
   Do not allow the back to arch at any time.

6. **REPETITIONS:** 2 sets of 10 reps.

NOTES

EXERCISE # 52
PELVIC LIFT

The pelvic lift is the same start position as the pelvic curl, except lifting higher.
This will also strengthen and tighten the buttocks.

1. EXERCISE:

i) After the curl has been achieved, continue
breathing out and peel the spine off the
floor until the hips are raised off the floor.
The lower back does not arch and no
pressure is felt in the spine.

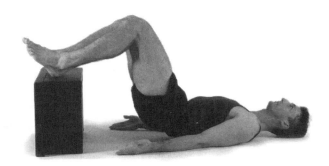

ii) All the work should still be controlled
from the abdominals.

iii) Breathe In and imprint the spine vertebra
at a time when releasing the position.

2. CARE:

i) Do not place any pressure on the heels. The knees should be hip distance apart and the knees at a
right angle above the navel when in the rest position.

ii) Remember to peel the spine off the floor and to imprint it back on. Do not peel the spine off any
higher than is comfortable and certainly not to where the back arches.

6. REPETITIONS: One set of ten reps.

NOTES

The Complete Guide to the Pilates Method

EXERCISE # 53 - 1
TEASER 1 - BASIC

1. **PREREQUISITE:** Hundreds (#31), PAC (#25), Roll-overs (#34).

2. **PURPOSE:** Abdominal strength through a continuous movement.

Figure i

3. **EXERCISE: Starting position:**
   Lie on your back with knees bent, arms above
   the head on the floor. Extend one leg into the air,
   keeping both knees at the same level (Figure i).

   i) Extend you hands, shoulder distance apart,
   in a line just above the **B-Line** and **Breathe
   Out** as you roll your spine off the mat in a
   long curve like the arch of a bow, neck long.

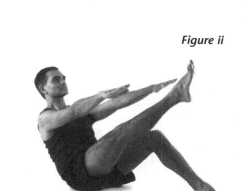

   ii) As you come up to the highest point, without
   any pressure on the feet, extend the fingers further
   to the line above the toes, without rounding the shoulders.

   iii) Breathe In and straighten the back, opening
   the chest, lift the ribs from the hips, sit tall on the
   sit bones (Figure ii).

Figure ii

   iv) Breathe Out as you lower yourself back to the
   mat, starting with a very small posterior pelvic tuck
   (or sink into the hips), keeping the back extended like
   the curve of a long bow, back to the stretch position.

   v) Do not rest. Keep all the muscles engaged and move
   immediately to the next repetition.

4. **KEY POINTS:**
   Flatten the ribs before the lift, so the line of the ribs and upper abdominals are flat throughout
   the movement.
   Shoulder blades to hips, lengthen the neck.
   Lift tall out of the hips as if you are trying to extend the lower back.
   Try to achieve the Greyhound's Stomach even while extending the back - this is a challenge!

5. **CARE:** If you feel the tops of the thighs overworking, do less repetitions or do some Quadriceps
   Stretches before continuing (Exercise # 13).

6. **REPETITIONS:** Up to 8 Teasers.

ADVANCED:
   Lie on your back with both feet resting lightly on a box or high chair, legs parallel and extended at
   approximately 45°, feet softly pointed. Arms above the head on the floor. Continue as in 3. i) above.

BREATHING SUMMARY:
   BO on the torso lift.
   BI back to the floor.

EXERCISE # 53 - II
TEASER II

1. PREREQUISITE: Teaser (Basic #53-I).

2. PURPOSE: Abdominal Strength, hip mobility; lower back stretch, hip flexor control.

3. EXERCISE: Starting Position: Sit tall on your sit bones, legs extended parallel, toes pointed. Arms at shoulder level, extended forward.

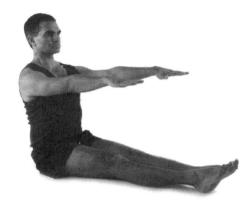

i) B-Line and **Breathe In**. Lean the torso back to a 45°angle as you raise legs into a V sit-up. Lift the legs level with your head (or as close as you can), balancing on your sit bones. See if you can touch your toes to your fingers, keeping the back, straight, shoulderblades to hips, neck long.

ii) Pause for a second, consolidating the strength of the abdominals and the firm lengthening of the torso. Squeeze the inner thighs.

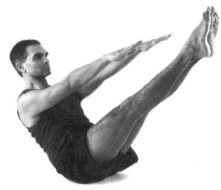

iii) Breathe Out as you lower the legs, extending through the toes to just off the floor back to the start position. Do not rest.

iv) Repeat.

4. KEY POINTS:

Keep the shoulders relaxed.
Keep the neck in line with the upper back.
Keep the ribs flat when the torso extends.
Stretch through the crown of the head and through the point of the toes.

5 & 6. CARE & REPITITIONS: See #53-I.

NOTES

EXERCISE # 53 - III
TEASER III

1. **PREREQUISITE:** Teaser (#52-II).

2. **PURPOSE:** Balance and Control.

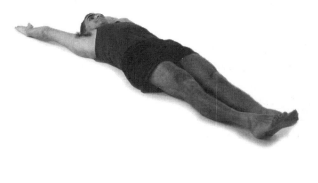

3. **EXERCISE: Starting position:**
   Lie on your back (supine), legs extended
   parallel, feet pointed. Arms extended through
   the fingertips above the head, shoulder width apart.

   i) B-Line and **Breathe Out** as you lift the legs,
   arms and torso in one movement into a V-sit-up
   position. Balance on your sit bones, reaching for
   the toes with the fingers. Keep the back as upright
   as possible (as if there were a rod in your spine).
   Keep the neck long.

   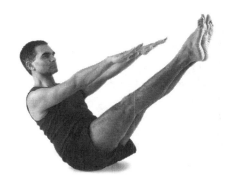

   ii) Breathe In as you slightly tuck the pelvis, contracting
   the abdominals and slowly elongate the torso, legs and arms
   back onto the mat at the same time, to the start position.

ADVANCED:
   At the end of lifting the legs, extend the arms up to
   the ceiling in line with your ears, shoulderblades to hips.
   Then continue with ii) above.

4. **KEY POINTS:** Same as Teaser (#53-I).

5. **CARE:** Same as Teaser (#53-I).

6. **REPETITIONS:** Up to ten reps.

NOTES

EXERCISE # 54
LEG PULL FRONT

1. **PREREQUISITE:** Hundreds (#31).

2. **PURPOSE:** Open the hip joints and strengthen the lower back and shoulders.

3. **EXERCISE: Starting position:**
   Assume a push-up position; arms locked, fingers pointing forward with the shoulders, hips and heels in a straight line.

   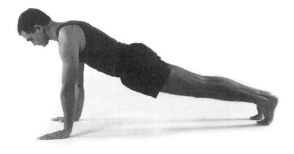

   i) B-Line with a slight tuck to help connect the lower abdominals. Keep the neck long in a straight line with the back. Press the heel into the floor as far as you can. Tighten the buttocks.

   ii) Breathe In as you lift the left leg, foot hard flexed, as high as you can to the ceiling (keep the knee joint locked) without allowing the hips to move or the back to arch.

   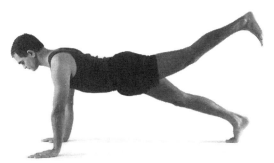

   iii) Breathe Out as you lower the leg to the floor, lengthen further through the heel. Touch the toe on the mat and repeat on the same leg.

   ADVANCED: At the top of the leg lift, do a double kick with an extra breath out. Point the foot as it touches the floor.

4. **KEY POINTS:** As you breathe in and extend the leg up, flatten the rib cage and tuck the pelvis.
   Consciously feel the abdominals tighten and support the entire body.
   Lengthen through the crown of the head in a straight line through the heels.
   B-Line and keep the abdominals continuously firm.
   Keep the balance of the toes between the joints of the big toe and the second toe.

5. **CARE:** Keep the elbows lengthened and locked. Do not hyper-extend as this may cause a strain at the elbow joint.

6. **REPETITIONS:** One set of 5 on each leg.

BREATHING SUMMARY:
   Breathe In as you lift the leg.
   Breathe Out as you lower the leg.

NOTES

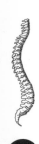

The Complete Guide to the Pilates Method

EXERCISE # 55
LEG PULL BACK

1. **PREREQUISITE:** Hamstring Stretches (#9-2), Quadriceps stretches (#13), Leg Pull Front (#54).

2. **PURPOSE:** Mobilize hip joints, stretch hamstrings, stabilize shoulders.

3. **EXERCISE: Starting position:**
   This is the reverse position to the push up.
   Chest facing the ceiling, extend the arms below
   the shoulders. Keep the shoulders, hips and heels
   in a straight line; toes pointed; chin to rib cage;
   pelvis slightly tucked under (posteriorly),
   shoulder blades to hips.

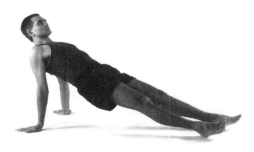

   i) B-Line and flex your right foot and **Breathe In** as
   you kick the leg to the ceiling (and past the vertical
   line if you can), pulling the abdominals in tighter.
   Keep the hips pressed to the ceiling, lift the chest
   to the ceiling, lengthen the back of the neck.
   Shoulders relaxed. Ribs to hips, abdominals firm.

   ii) Point the foot and **Breathe Out** as you slowly
   lower the leg to the floor.

   iii) Touch lightly on the floor and kick the same
   leg again.

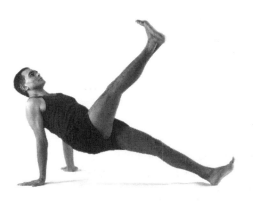

   ADVANCED: At the top of the kick do a double kick
   and a double breath in.

4. **KEY POINTS:** Keep the pelvis lifted up as the leg kicks up.
   Elongate the head and neck out of the shoulders.
   Ensure the pressure on the supporting leg is in the centre of the heel.

5. **CARE:** Imagine there is a rod from the centre top of the shoulders to the tailbone and another
   across the shoulders.
   Avoid hyper-extending the elbows.

6. **REPETITIONS:** 5 kicks on each leg.

BREATHING SUMMARY:
   Breathe In on the kick up.
   Breathe Out on the return.

NOTES

EXERCISE # 56
SIDE KICK II

1. **PREREQUISITES:** Start stretches, Hundreds (# 31), Side Kick-I (#49).

2. **PURPOSE:** Mobilize the hips, stretch the thigh, strengthen the lower back.

3. **EXERCISE: Starting position:**
   Lie on the floor on you right side, place your head in the right hand.

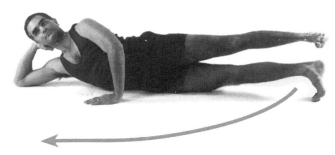

   i) Keeping your legs straight, bring them slightly forward, top leg parallel and both feet flexed, bottom leg turned out with toe pressed into the floor. Lengthening through the heels.
   Lift the left leg slightly to hip level, keep the foot flexed and **B-Line**.

   ii) Take a deep **Breath In** as you kick the leg forward as far as you can, pressing through the heel.
   Keep the spine straight.
   At the end of the kick, do a further, smaller kick inhaling an extra breath to expand the lungs further.

   iii) Point your foot and **Breathe Out** as you kick your leg back in a sweeping motion. As the top leg sweeps behind the straight line of the body, raise the torso up onto the right elbow, creating a large gap under your right armpit.

   iv) Flex the foot and press through the heel for the next kick forward.
   As the leg kicks forward again, lean back slightly to reduce the gap under the armpit, keeping the back as straight as possible and flatten the rib cage.

4. **KEY POINTS:** Stabilize your centre and, as if your hip were the centre of a circle, lengthen through the heel and toe reaching past the outer rim of the circle.
   Keep the shoulders stable and chin lifted.
   Lengthen through the crown of the head.
   To keep the top hip directly above the bottom one, create a small gap between the waist and the floor.

5. **CARE:** If any strain is felt in the back, discontinue the exercise.
   If you feel the hip bone on the mat, place a flat cushion under the hip.

6. **REPETITIONS:** 10 kicks each side.

BREATHING SUMMARY:
   Breathe In kick forward, extra breath in at the stretch.
   Breathe Out kick back.

ADVANCED: Starting position:
   Place the left hand behind your head, elbow to the ceiling in line with the body.

NOTES

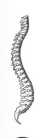

EXERCISE # 57
BOOMERANG

1. **PREREQUISITE:** Teaser (#53-II), Roll-over (#34).

2. **PURPOSE:** Control, mobilization of spine, shoulders and hips, stretch hamstrings.

3. **EXERCISE: Starting position:**
B-Line and sit upright on the floor with an imaginary rod up your spine, palms on the floor by the hips, legs extended forward locked at the knee joint with the right ankle crossed over the left.

i) Tuck the pelvis slightly, take a deep **Breathe Out** as you sink into your hips and roll back, drawing the thighs to the ribs into a roll-over till the feet almost touch the mat. Lengthen the neck and roll only to the top of the shoulders (Figure i).

Figure i

ii) At this point, squeezing the inner thighs, quickly cross the legs the other way (left over right).

iii) Breathe In as you roll forward extending your arms off the floor, out to the sides and behind your back. Try to hold the left hand with the right, elbows locked and continue to extend the hands behind you and up towards the ceiling.

iv) Balance on your sit bones for 3 seconds with the legs 30cm off the floor, spine erect, legs straight (Figure ii).

Figure ii

v) Breathe Out as you continue the roll forward lengthening your chest towards your knees and head towards your feet, extended hands pressing to the ceiling (Figure iii).

Figure iii

vi) Breathe In as you release the hands and stretch them around in a circle to the ceiling, rotating the shoulder joints, at the same time imprint the torso into the upright sitting position, hands by the hips.

4. **KEY POINTS:** The entire movement centres around contracted and controlled abdominal strength, precision and flowing movement.

5. **CARE:** Roll back only on to the tops of the shoulders. Keep the shoulder blades to the hips and neck straight and long when clasping the hands behind the back.

6. **REPETITIONS:** One set of up to 8 complete movements.

BREATHING SUMMARY:
Breathe In sit tall.
Breathe Out roll over.
Breathe In roll up to balance.
Hold for three seconds.
Breathe Out roll and reach chest to knees.
Breathe In extend to upright.

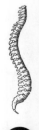

EXERCISE # 58
SEAL

1. **PREREQUISITE:** Roll-overs (#34).

2. **PURPOSE:** Control, stretch the spine.

3. **EXERCISE: Starting position:** Sit tall on the mat, knees bent and open, elbows placed on the inside of the thighs, forearms under the calves and holding onto the front of the ankles, arms straight. Soles of the feet together, heels off the mat and toes lightly touching.

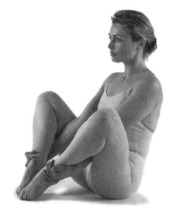

   i) B-Line and **Breathe Out** as you tuck the pelvis to start to roll the spine and continue to smoothly roll over onto the top of the shoulders until the heels are 5cms of the mat.

   ii) Balancing in this position, open the feet 20cms and clap them together 3 times.

   iii) Breathe In as you roll into the start position, straightening the spine at the top of the roll, toes just off the mat, clap the soles of the feet 3 times.

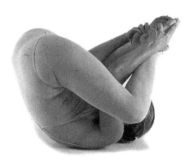

4. **KEY POINTS:** Keep the neck long.
   Ribs to hips on the roll back.
   When balancing on the shoulders, keep the abdominals hollow and firm.

5. **CARE:** Keep the shoulderblades to the hips to avoid neck strain.

6. **REPETITIONS:** One set of up to 8 reps.

BREATHING SUMMARY:
   Breathe In sit in a continuous 'C' curve.
   Breathe Out roll back.
   Hold for the 3 claps.
   Breathe In on the roll up sitting tall.

NOTES

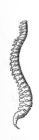

The Complete Guide to the Pilates Method

EXERCISE # 59
CONTROL BALANCE

1. **PREREQUISITE:** Roll Overs (#34).

2. **PURPOSE:** Control, balance and abdominal strength.

3. **EXERCISE: Starting position:**
   Lie on your back with the arms above your head on the floor,
   legs are vertical and parallel.

   i) B-Line and **Breathe Out** as you roll over until the toes touch
   the mat, tailbone to ceiling.
   Hold onto the right ankle with both hands.

   ii) Breathe In as you extend the left leg to the ceiling, turned out and
   foot pointed, past the vertical line of the hip, extending through the toes.
   Extend the spine as upright as possible, pressing the tailbone to the
   ceiling and the toes of the right foot into the floor above your head.

   iii) Breathe In as you release the right ankle, smoothly scissors
   the legs, keeping the torso and legs under control.
   The tailbone remains lengthened to the ceiling.

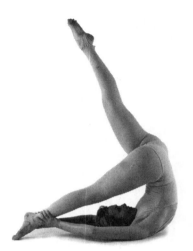

   iv) Breathe Out as you extend the right leg to the ceiling, turned out and pointed. Holding onto the left
   ankle, leg parallel, press the toe into the mat and lenghening through the heel.

4. **KEY POINTS:** By pressing the heel to the mat a better stretch up the back of the leg is achieved.
   Keep the extended leg to the ceiling, locked at the knee joint.
   Consciously think of releasing the front of the thigh.

5. **CARE:** Keep the shoulders open and on the mat, neck lengthened.
   This will provide more stability for the movement.
   Keep the abdominals hollow and the back straight.

6. **REPETITIONS:** One set of 6 extensions on each leg.

BREATHING SUMMERY:
   Breathe Out as the leg extends to the ceiling.
   Breathe In as the legs change direction.

NOTES

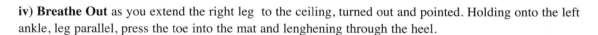

MORE ADVANCED ROUTINE

EXERCISE # 60
HUNDREDS - LOWER & RAISE

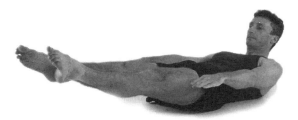

1. **PREREQUISITE:** Hundreds (#31).

2. **PURPOSE:** Greater abdominal strength with increased body extension.

3. **EXERCISE:** Same **start position** as Hundreds (#31). Keep the feet pointed and turned out.

   i) B-Line and **Breathe Out** as you lower the legs down to eye level (or the most comfortable position) for a 5 second count, at the same time still trying to lift your buttocks off the floor for stronger, lower abdominal connection!

   ii) Point the feet, **B-Line** harder and, **Breathe In** as you raise the legs back to the vertical position squeezing the inner thighs.

4. **KEY POINTS:** Same as those in the Hundreds (#31) as well as:

   i) When lowering the legs, squeeze the inner thighs and allow the abdominal muscles to slowly 'release' to allow the legs to lower without the back arching.

   ii) Then anchor the abdominals before lifting the legs, imagine the hips drawing to the ribs; the contraction of the abdominals is what floats the legs back to the vertical position; squeezing the inner thighs.

   iii) As the legs are lowered be sure not to lower the head and shoulders as this will arch the back (looking in a mirror at the stability of the torso may help).

5. **CARE:** If, after lowering or raising the legs, you feel as if the abdominals have 'had enough', return to the rest position.

6. **REPETITIONS:** 2 sets of ten, 5 seconds rest between each set.

NOTES

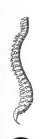

EXERCISE #61
ROLL OVER - BENT LEGS

1. **PREREQUISITE:** Roll-over straight legs (#34), Rolling (#37).

2. **PURPOSE:** To connect the deeper abdominal muscles, especially in the lower abdominal section.

3. **EXERCISE: Starting position:**
Lie on the floor with your back flat, knees bent to
the chest and open shoulder distance, ankles crossed.

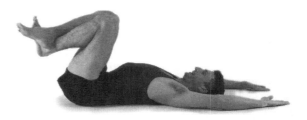

i) B-Line and, attempting to keep the heels as close
as you can to your buttocks, **Breathe Out** as you roll
the hips off the floor to your ribs. Draw the knees
close to your chest and in towards your armpits.

ii) Roll onto the shoulders only, lengthen your neck.

iii) Breathe into your upper back as you hold the position.

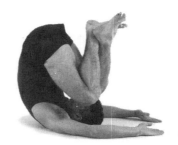

iv) Breathe Out as you <u>slowly</u> roll back, imprinting your spine
onto the floor, slowly release the abdominals to prevent the
head and shoulders lifting off the floor.

4. **KEY POINTS:** If you are unable to perform the exercise
with the heels to the tailbone, lengthen the legs until more
control is attained.
It is on the roll down that you will feel the lower abdominals connecting.
Continue the repetitions without any rest.
Keep the thighs close to the body at all times.

5. **CARE:** Roll onto the shoulders only, not the neck.
Start this exercise with your legs long and bent, ankles crossed. As you become more proficient,
keep the heels closer to the tailbone.
The last 25% of the exercise, on the release, is the most challenging to control.

6. **REPETITIONS:** one set of 10, ankles crossed each way after each roll.

NOTES

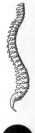

EXERCISE # 62
PENDULUM

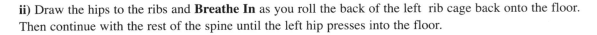

1. **PREREQUISITE:** Corkscrew (#47-II).

2. **PURPOSE:** Strengthen the obliques and abdominals, mobilize
   and strengthen the spine.

3. **EXERCISE: Starting position:**
   Lie on your back on the floor, legs straight to the ceiling,
   turned out and feet pointed. Arms above the head, elbows
   bent and pressed into the mat, hands slightly wider than
   shoulder distance.
   (Basic version is with hands by the sides as in the photo).

   i) B-Line and keeping the feet together, **Breathe Out**
   as your legs go over to the right in line with your navel,
   The left hip lifts off the floor.
   Keep the shoulder blades and elbows pressed into the mat.

   ii) Draw the hips to the ribs and **Breathe In** as you roll the back of the left rib cage back onto the floor.
   Then continue with the rest of the spine until the left hip presses into the floor.

   iii) Keep moving to the other side without stopping.
   Turn the head in the opposite direction to the legs.

4. **KEY POINTS:** Keep the legs turned out, especially when returning to the vertical position.
   Release the opposite chest muscle to allow the shoulder to stay on the mat.
   If there is too much pressure on the arms to raise the legs back to the vertical position, then the legs
   have gone over too far.
   When over to the side, draw the legs up to the elbow to keep the abdominals connected and prevent the
   back from arching.
   Keep the toes in line with the navel .

   As more control develops, take the legs further over to the sides to several centimeters off the floor without
   the shoulder blades lifting at all! Well done if you are able to do this without straining!

5. **REPETITIONS:** One set, 10 each side alternating.

NOTES

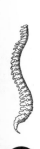

EXERCISE # 63
NECK PULL

1. **PREREQUISITES:** Hundred (#60), Curls (#25) with straight legs.

2. **PURPOSE:** To improve abdominal control and strength.

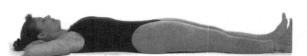

Figure i

3. **EXERCISE: Starting position:**
   Lie on your back on the floor, legs extended
   15 cm apart in front of you; feet flexed,
   knees pressed into the floor.
   Place your hands behind your head, fingers
   interlocked, elbows on the mat (Figure i).

   i) B-Line and **Breathe In** as you raise the head and
   shoulders off the mat, keeping the elbows behind the
   ears, as if a bar is passing in front of the elbows and
   behind the head (Figure ii).

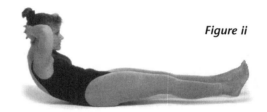

Figure ii

   ii) Breathe Out as you curl forward, contracting the ribs
   to the hips, zipping up the stomach. Reach forward as far
   as you can, trying to extend your chest to your knees.

   iii) Breathe In as you imprint your spine up an imaginary
   wall into the upright position.
   Lift the ribs out of the hips without hunching the shoulders
   (Figure iii).

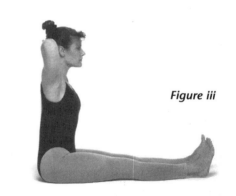

Figure iii

   iv) Breathe Out as you sink into the hips, tucking the pelvis
   to connect the lower abdominals, press through the heels and
   imprint your spine on the mat, keeping the ribs to the hips
   until the shoulderblades rest on the mat (Figure ii).

   v) Extend the neck onto the mat keeping the **B-Line**.

4. **KEY POINTS:** Zip up the stomach before you start to lift the head.
   Keep the elbows open.
   Keep the shoulderblades to the hips.
   Peel your spine off the mat.

5. **CARE:** Breathe Out 75% of your capacity in the first 25% of the movements up or down.
   Flatten the ribs to the floor before rolling the shoulders off the mat.
   Keep the chin slightly off the chest.
   Do not pull on the neck, elbows always wide open!

6. **REPETITIONS:** One set of up to 10.

BREATHING SUMMARY:
   Breathe In as the head and shoulders lift upright.
   Breathe Out as you roll up and forward.
   Breathe In as you imprint to the vertical.
   Breathe Out as you roll down.

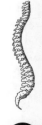

EXERCISE # 64
JACKNIFE

1. **PREREQUISITE:** Roll-over (#61), Hundred (#70), Curls (#25) with straight legs.

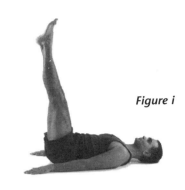

Figure i

2. **PURPOSE:** Stretch the spine, stretch the neck, abdominal control.

3. **EXERCISE: Starting position:** Lie on your back, palms down, legs extended vertically, toes pointed and parallel (Figure i).

   i) Breathe Out as you roll over onto the shoulders without allowing the legs to lower to the floor (Figure ii).

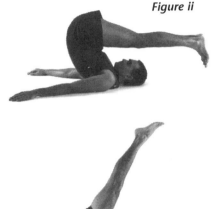

Figure ii

   ii) Immediately lengthen the legs to a vertical position as if the body were in a straight line to the ceiling.
Extend through the toes, squeeze the inner thighs and hold the buttocks firmly. Press your hips towards a straight line above your eyes (Figure iii).

   iii) Balance and hold the position for the **Breathe In**.

   iv) Breathe Out as you slowly imprint your spine on the mat, trying the keep you feet above your eyes until the hips have lengthened away from the ribs and pressed into the mat (Figure iv).

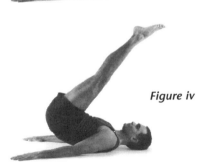

Figure iii

   v) Breathe In as you lower the legs towards the floor to a level where the back remains flat (**B-Line**).

   vi) Repeat.

4. **KEY POINTS:** Keep the shoulders relaxed, without much pressure into the hands.
The jacknife over is a fast movement, and slowly down.
Total focus on flat, strong abdominals is required at all times.

Figure iv

5. **CARE:** Keep the neck as long as possible.
Avoid this exercise unless you feel 100% confident that you can control the movement 100%.
The movement must be smooth and elegant throughout.

6. **REPETITIONS:** One set of up to 8 reps.

BREATHING SUMMARY:
   Breathe Out as you jacknife over and up to vertical.
   Balance and Breathe In into the back.
   Breathe Out on the roll down.

NOTES

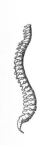

EXERCISE # 65
SCISSORS

1. **PREREQUISITES:** Hundreds (#31), Roll-overs (#61), Jacknife (#64).

2. **PURPOSE:** Abdominal control, stretch the upper back and neck. mobilize the hips, hip flexor stretch.

3. **EXERCISE: Starting position:** Lie on your back with your legs extended, hands by your sides, palms down.

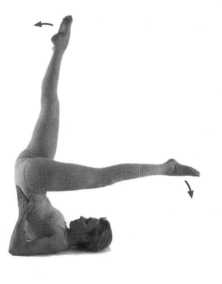

   i) B-Line and **Breathe Out** as you do a jacknife (Exercise # 64) to the ceiling and in the vertical position place your hands into the small of your back to support your hips in an upright position; elbows pressed on the mat and close to each other.

   ii) Keeping the knees locked, toes pointed and the buttocks held firmly, **Breathe Out** as you stretch the right leg away from your head past the point of the elbows towards the floor.
   At the same time lower and stretch the left leg past your head so the left knee is in line with your eyes. (Photo)

   iii) Breathe In as you bring both legs to the vertical position, squeezing the inner thighs, smoothly change over.

   iv) Breathe Out as you change legs.

4. **KEY POINTS:** As the leg stretches past the point of the elbows (and the vertical line to the ceiling), draw the hip bones to the rib cage.
   You will feel the abdominals connect more, this will minimize any tendancy to arch the back.
   A triangle of your hands, elbows and shoulders provides the infrastructure for the position of the movement.
   The control is always firmly from the centre with the ribs flat.

5. **CARE:** Keep the neck relaxed and lengthened.
   The hand should be lightly supporting the lower back, not providing the main support.
   The chin should be slightly off the chest so the breathing can flow easily.

6. **REPETITIONS:** One set of 5 each side

BREATHING SUMMARY:
   Breathe Out on the scissors.
   Breathe In on the close of the legs.

ADVANCED VERSION: Perform the scissors more rapidly, Breathe In for 2 scissors and Breathe Out for 2 scissors. IN IN (stretch, stretch) OUT OUT (stretch, stretch).

NOTES

EXERCISE # 66
BICYCLE

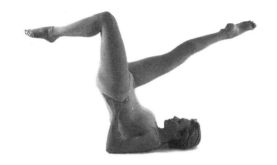

1. **PREREQUISITE:** Scissors (#65).

2. **PURPOSE:** Mobilize hip joints, keep abdominals long and strong, stretch hip flexors, stabilize the pelvic area.

3. **EXERCISE: Starting position:**
   The start position is the same as for the Scissors.
   Once you have attained the upright position then:

   i) **B-Line** and **Breathe Out** as you extend the left leg past the point of the elbows and bend the knee to reach the toes towards the floor (photo).

   ii) **Breathe In**, the left knee is drawn towards eye level and extended to the ceiling as the right leg extends past the point of the elbows and down to the floor, while the left foot extends to the ceiling with the knee above the eyes.

   The action is that of pedaling a bicycle (hence, the name).

4. **KEY POINTS:** Consciously stretch the front of the thigh as you extend the leg and bend the knee, pointing the toe to the floor.
   Imagine the hip to the rib of the thigh being stretched.
   As the knee draws towards eye level, keep the abdominals firm.
   The knee is not drawn towards the face or chest; the cycling action is kept away from the chest.

5. **CARE:** As the foot extends to the floor, keep any excessive pressure off the hands as this will place more pressure into the lower back.

6. **REPETITIONS:** One set of 5 cycling motions with each leg.

BREATHING SUMMARY:
   Breathe Out as the leg stretches for the floor.
   Breathe In for the cycle movement.

NOTES

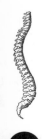

144

EXERCISE # 67
SHOULDER BRIDGE

1. **PREREQUISITE:** Hundreds (#31).

2. **PURPOSE:** Extend the lower back while providing support for the abdominals, Stretch the hip flexors.

3. **EXERCISE: Starting position:** Lie on your back with the knees bent, feet parallel, hands by your sides.

    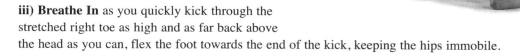

    i) B-Line and **Breathe Out** as you curl the hips up from the mat, lengthen the neck and support the back by placing one hand under each hip, elbows under the hands, feet firmly pressed into the mat.

    ii) Breathe Out as you point the right foot and stretch it as close to the floor as you can until the leg is straight, knee locked.

    iii) Breathe In as you quickly kick through the stretched right toe as high and as far back above the head as you can, flex the foot towards the end of the kick, keeping the hips immobile.

    iv) Breathe Out as you slowly lower the right leg to the floor with the flexed foot. Press the heel as far as you can to the ground then point the foot and repeat.

4. **KEY POINTS:** Keep the buttocks gently held together.
    The shoulders, elbows and feet support the position.
    The abdominals are firmly held, with ribs to hips.
    When lowering the leg, stretch the top of the thigh, zip up the stomach and imagine you are tucking the pelvis under to open the lower back.

5. **CARE:** Keep the lower back as open as possible, especially when the leg lowers to the floor.
    B-Line firmly.

6. **REPETITIONS:** 5 kicks on the right leg, 5 kicks on the left.

BREATHING SUMMARY:
    Breathe Out as you stretch to the floor.
    Breathe In as you kick.
    Breathe Out as you lower and stretch the leg.

NOTES

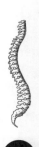

EXERCISE # 68
CAN CAN

1. **PREREQUISITES:** Hundreds (#31), Side to Side (#23).

2. **PURPOSE:** Mobilize the lower back and hips.

3. **EXERCISE: Starting Position:** Sit upright with your hands behind you on the floor, elbows straight. Feet close to your bottom, toes pointed and touching the floor. Knees together.

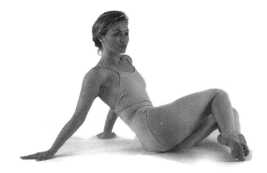

   i) **B-Line** and **Breathing Out** let both knees lower to the floor to the left. The right buttock may raise off the floor.

   ii) **B-Line** harder and **Breathing In**, raise both knees back to the start position by drawing the **front** of the right hip to the floor.

   iii) Repeat to the other side, gradually getting the knees closer to the floor each time.

4. **KEY POINTS:** Keep the shoulders and upper torso as still as possible. On each movement to the side feel the lower back on that side opening. Squeeze the inner thighs.

5. **CARE:** If any twinge or strain is felt in the lower back, do not lower the knees too far to the side.

6. **REPETITIONS:** 10 to each side.

NOTES

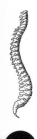

The Complete Guide to the Pilates Method

EXERCISE 68 - I
CAN CAN EXTENSION

This is the advanced version of the Can Can above with the following addition:

1. **PREREQUISITES:** Can Can (# 68).

2. **PURPOSE:** Mobilize and strengthen lower back, hips and lower abdominals.

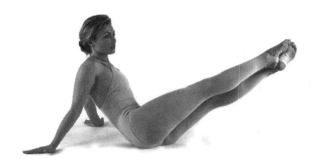

3. **EXERCISE: Starting position:**
   As in Can Can (#68).

   i) After lowering the knees to the side (less than your normal distance), **B-Line** and **Breathe In** as you then extend the legs (still keeping them together) into the air.

   ii) Breathe Out as you draw the heels back to your tailbone and continue as in Can Can to the other side.

4. **KEY POINTS:** Try not to lean back as the legs extend. Keep the arms and back as straight as possible.

5. **CARE:** The Quadriceps may feel as if they are gripping on the extension, this will gradually ease. Stop at a comfortable number of repetitions if you unable to complete 10.

6. **REPETITIONS:** 10 each side.

NOTES

EXERCISE # 69
HIP CIRCLES

This is similar to the Advanced Corkscrew in a seated position.

1. **PREREQUISITE:** Corkscrew (#47-II) Pendulum (#62), Can Can (#68-I).

2. **PURPOSE:** Abdominal and hip flexor strength, hip joint mobility, lower back mobility.

3. **EXERCISE: Starting position:**
   Sit upright on the mat. Keeping your spine as straight as possible, lean back with your hands behind you to a 45° angle.
   Hands wide and elbows locked.

   i) B-Line and bend your knees to the chest and extend them to the ceiling, feet pointed. Squeeze the inner thighs.

   ii) Breathe Out as you swing the legs around in a circle to the right, down to just off the mat and swing them around to the left.

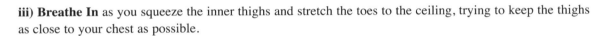

Legs together

   iii) Breathe In as you squeeze the inner thighs and stretch the toes to the ceiling, trying to keep the thighs as close to your chest as possible.

   iv) Repeat in the other direction.

4. **KEY POINTS:**
   Lengthen the neck out of the shoulders, as if someone is lengthening you up from the crown of your head.
   Keep the chest open and B-Line at all times.
   Zip up the stomach as the legs raise up to the ceiling.
   Keep the hips as square as you can. The hips will slightly raise off the floor as you go to the sides.
   As the legs lower to the floor, flatten the ribs to the hips keeping the spine long.
   Lengthen through the toes.

5. **CARE:** If you feel the exercise strongly in the wrists or shoulders, discontinue the exercise.
   Do not hunch the shoulders.

6. **REPETITIONS:** Up to 5 Hip Circles in each direction.

BREATHINGSUMMARY:
   Breathe Out on the lower part of the circle.
   Breathe In as you raise the legs to the ceiling.

NOTES

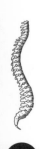

EXERCISE # 70
HELICOPTER HUNDREDS

1. **PREREQUISITE:** Hundreds (#31).

2. **PURPOSE:** Strengthen the abdominals, mobilize the hip joints.

3. **EXERCISE: Starting position:**
Lie on your back on the floor, knees to chest,
hands on ankles.

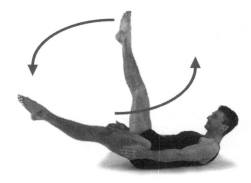

i) **B-Line** and **Breathe Out** as you contract
forward, arms extended just off the floor past
the hips; legs vertical, feet pointed and turned out.

ii) Scissor (or split) the legs, left leg to the ceiling and right
leg to the floor, then **Breathe In** as you take the legs around,
in opposite directions away from the body, in a circle, keeping
the legs turned out and feet pointed. The right leg opens to the
side and comes up to the vertical position, the left leg opens to
the side and lowers to just off the floor.

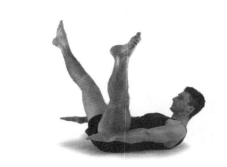

iii) **Breathe Out** scissor the legs.

iv) Repeat five times in each direction.

4. **KEY POINTS:** Lengthen out of the hip sockets as much as
possible maintaining your turnout.
Focus on the inner thigh (adductor) muscles to make the circle.

5. **CARE:** If the hips joints 'click' either:
   a) lengthen out of the hip joints further
   b) reduced the range of movement of the circle or
   c) reduce the turnout of the leg.

6. **REPETITIONS:** Repeat 5 times, then change direction.

BREATHING SUMMARY:
Breathe Out as you lower 'split' the legs.
Breathe In as you circle the legs.

NOTES

EXERCISE # 71
LYING TORSO STRETCH

1. **PREREQUISITES:** Side to side.

2. **PURPOSE:** This is a cooling down stretch. It mobilizes the mid-, upper-back and shoulders and releases tension in the lower back.

3. **EXERCISE: Starting position:** Lying on your right side, straighten the right leg and bend the left leg so it is lying on the floor in front of you, left heel touching right knee. The right arm is lengthened in front of the chest, palm up. The left arm is stretched out in front of the chest, reaching as far as possible through the fingertips, past the right hand, the left shoulder is also leaning forward.

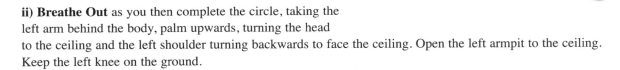

   i) B-Line and **Breathe In** as you scrape the floor with the fingers of the left hand making a circle until the arm is above the head.

   ii) Breathe Out as you then complete the circle, taking the left arm behind the body, palm upwards, turning the head to the ceiling and the left shoulder turning backwards to face the ceiling. Open the left armpit to the ceiling. Keep the left knee on the ground.

   iii) Complete the circle by taking the left hand towards the right foot and forward in front of the chest to the starting position.

4. **KEY POINTS:** As the shoulder loosens and the upper back becomes more flexible, the circling hand may eventually touch the floor for the movement.

   As the arm extends behind the body, lengthen the entire body from the toes of the lower leg through the fingertips of the circling arm.

   If you feel a particular point during the stretch where the muscles feel tight, stay in that position for several seconds to release the tension before continuing.

5. **CARE:**
   Do not try to force the top shoulder down to the floor. Allow the body to release into the stretch gradually.

6. **REPETITIONS:** One set of 10 reps. 5 circles in each direction.

NOTES

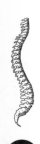

EXERCISE # 72
STANDING SIDE STRETCHES

1. PREREQUISITES: Nil.

2. PURPOSE: To stretch the muscles down the side of the body from the armpit to the hip.

3. EXERCISE: Starting position: Stand to the side of the frame of a doorway about 30cms away from the edge of the frame so it is on your right hand side.
Hold onto the door frame with the right hand just below hip level. Take the left hand over the head and hold onto the frame at approximately forehead level.

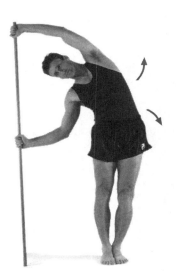

i) Breathe Out and stretch the body away from the frame as far as possible. Straighten the top arm. Press the left hip to the floor and the left lower ribs to the ceiling. Turn the armpit towards the ceiling for a much greater stretch of the muscle near the shoulder blade (latissimus dorsi).

ii) Breathe In without moving, Breathe Out and stretch a little further.

iii) After 5 breaths/stretches, B-Line harder and use the abdominals to return to the upright position. Do not use the arms.
Change sides and repeat the movement.

ADVANCED:
To create a greater stretch, press the right hand against the frame to increase the effectiveness of the stretch, without hunching the right shoulder.

4. KEY POINTS: Relax the inside shoulder.
Allow the head to relax under the right arm, looking straight ahead.

5. CARE: After stretching to the side, turn the hips slightly in (outside hip slightly in front of inside hip) to avoid any pressure in the back.
It the lower back feels tight during the exercise, tuck the pelvis under and this will open up the lower back.
A stretch may also be felt just above the hip in the lower back area.

6. REPETITIONS: 2 sets of 10 breaths in and out per side, alternating after each five.
Use the B-Line and not the arms when coming to the upright position after the 10 breaths.

EXERCISE # 72 - I

ADVANCED: Follow all instructions for Exercise # 72 and:

3. EXERCISE

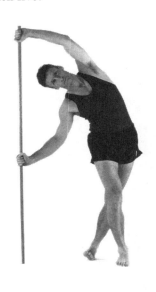

i) After position 72-3i) above, place the left leg behind the right leg on the outside edge of the left heel. Bend the right leg and continue as above. This will give a greater stretch to the top outside of the hip.

EXERCISE # 73
CAT STRETCH

1. **PREREQUISITES:** Nil.

2. **PURPOSE:** Flexion mobility for the spine.

3. **EXERCISE: Starting position:** Kneel on all fours, knees and hands shoulder distance apart. Head relaxed in line with the spine.

   i) **Breath Out** as you slowly draw the head to the groin while pressing the spine to the ceiling.

   ii) **Breathe In** as you release the ribs away from the hips until the spine is horizontal to the floor. *Lengthen* the hips away from the ribs.

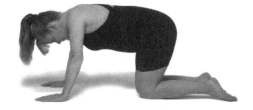

4. **KEY POINTS:** Attempt to draw your nose to your B-Line and your hips to your ribs in the same movement. This will stretch the cervical, thoracic and lumbar areas of the spine.

5. **CARE:** If there is too much mobility in the upper back, concentrate more on drawing the hips to the ribs. This exercise is great for pregnant women (photo) as it stretches the tight lower back muscles.

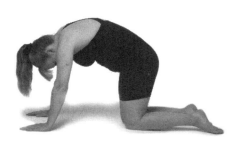

6. **REPETITIONS:** 10 stretches.

NOTES

EXERCISE # 74
ROCKING

1. **PREREQUISITE:** Strong back required! Quadriceps (#13-lunge), Swan II (#42-I).

2. **PURPOSE:** Control and stretch the front (anterior) part of the body, work and strengthen the back muscles.

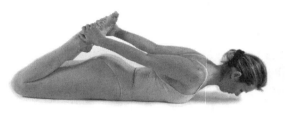

3. **EXERCISE: Starting position:**
   Lie prone on the mat and drawing the heels to your buttocks, knees shoulder width apart, feet slightly closer; reach behind you and hold the outsides of the feet with your hands. Keep the shoulder blades to the hips and extend the crown of the head towards the line of the toes.

   i) B-Line and **Breathing Out**, roll forward onto the chest, keeping your chin off the floor.

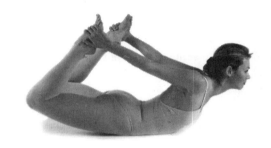

   ii) Breathe In as you rock backwards as hard as you can, opening the chest and lift it off the mat. Keep the buttocks tight.

   iii) Breathe Out and repeat **i)** above.

4. **KEY POINTS:** Think of your spine like the curved legs of a rocking chair. Rock and elongate through the tips of the knees and the top of the chest.
   Keep the spine as long and **open** as possible.
   Flatten the rib cage on the roll forward so it does not poke into the mat.
   Keep the abdominals hollow and firm.

5. **CARE:** If the back feels any pressure - stop.
   Keep the shoulders open and down to the hips.

6. **REPETITIONS:** One set of up to 8 rocking movements.

BREATHING SUMMARY:
   Breathe Out rolling forward.
   Breathe In rolling onto the thighs.

NOTES

EXERCISE # 75 - I
TWIST I

1. **PREREQUISITE:** Hamstring stretches (#10), Pendulum (#62).

2. **PURPOSE:** Rotation for the spine, open the lower back,
   mobilizes and strengthen the shoulder girdle.

3. **EXERCISE: Starting position:**
   Sit partially on your right hip, knees towards the chest, left ankle
   over right with the sole of the left foot flat on the mat toes pointing
   forward, heels close to the tailbone. With the right arm close to the
   right hip, palm pressed into the mat pointed slightly forward.
   Lean slightly forward over the hand. Left hand relaxed on left ankle.

   i) B-Line and **Breathe In** as you lift your tailbone to the ceiling
   as if you were being lifted by a piece of string attached to this
   point. The balance control is from the palm of the right hand
   and sole of the left foot.

   ii) As the tailbone extends upwards, reach through the
   fingertips of the left hand away from the body, in a smooth
   arc up to the ceiling and over towards the floor close to the
   left ear. The crown of the head and the fingers of the left
   hand should be reaching to the mat.

   iii) Breathe In as you reverse the movement, connecting
   the abdominals as if you are still being pulled by the tailbone
   to the ceiling. Extend the left arm as if you are drawing
   a line on the ceiling with your fingertips.

4. **KEY POINTS:** Reach the fingers of the moving arm, with the elbow joint unlocked, as if you want to
   touch the ceiling in both directions.
   Lift the tailbone as high as you can, trying to straighten the spine, keeping the abdominals hollow.
   Shoulder blades to hips.
   The movement is smooth and flowing as if being performed by a ballet dancer.

5. **CARE:** The balance comes from the following:
   i) Place equal pressure on the heel of the hand as well as the fingertips of the right hand, extending the
   fingers on the mat.
   ii) Place equal pressure on the tripod of the left foot.
   The control emanates from the abdominals and the strength of the right shoulder.

6. **REPETITIONS:** One set of 5 each side.

BREATHING SUMMARY:
   Breathe In on the extension to the ceiling.
   Breathe Out on the return to the mat.

NOTES

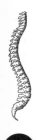

The Complete Guide to the Pilates Method

EXERCISE # 75 - II
TWIST II

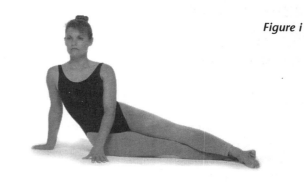

Figure i

1. **PREREQUISITE:** Twist I (#75-I).

2. **PURPOSE:** Advanced balance and control.

3. **EXERCISE: Starting position:**
   Sit upright on the mat, legs extended; place the right
   hand on the floor slightly behind you and lean over
   onto the right hip so your torso faces away from the
   upright position. Cross the left leg on top of the right
   leg. Left hand relaxed on the floor in front of the thigh.
   (Figure i).

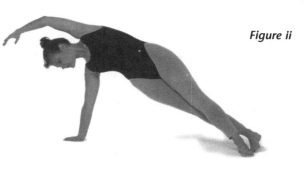

Figure ii

   i) B-Line and **Breathe In** as you lift the left hip bone
   vertically as if it is attached to a string drawing
   upwards. The control point is from the placement of
   the left sole as much into the floor as possible.
   Squeeze the inner thighs.
   ii) As the movement begins, extend the left hand
   (elbow unlocked) towards the left foot, then draw
   a line to the ceiling and over towards a point above
   the left ear. Maintain absolute control (Figure ii).
   iii) Breathe In as you rotate only the torso to face the
   floor by rotating the left shoulder blade towards the
   right hand. Feel the obliques muscles on both sides
   connect. Keep the left arm in line with the ear, left
   shoulder blade to left hip.
   iv) Breathe In as you rotate the torso back and
   continue as if you are opening your chest to the
   ceiling. The obliques and the abdominals are still
   strongly connected. Stretch the top of the thighs.
   (Figure iii)
   v) Breathe Out as you return to the start, reversing
   the movements in **ii)** and **i)**.

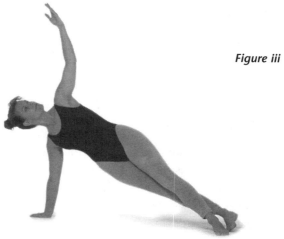

Figure iii

4. **KEY POINTS:** When lifting the hip to the ceiling a straight line should be achieved, as if along a pole
   from the feet, tailbone, spine and crown of the head.
   Keep the pelvis tucked under for better lower abdominal connection (this is not usually visually apparent.
   It is the internal connection that is more important).

5. **CARE:** Maintain careful, smooth control on the rotation of the torso.
   It is a precise movement that requires every fibre of the body to be active and all your concentration
   to be focused for the best result.

6. **REPETITIONS:** One set up to 5 Twists on each side.

BREATHING SUMMARY:
   Breathe In on the lift.
   Breathe Out rotate to the floor.
   Breathe In rotate to the ceiling.
   Breathe Out return to start.

FURTHER SPECIFIC EXERCISES

EXERCISE # 76
OBLIQUE CURLS

1. **PREREQUISITE:** Perfect Abdominal Curl (# 25).

2. **PURPOSE:** To strengthen the obliques. This is an advanced exercise.

3. **EXERCISE:** In essence, this exercise is the same as the Curls but with a twist.
   Starting position: Lie on the floor with knees bent (right angle at knee joint), contract forward with hands behind the head, elbows open.

   i) **Breathe Out** and Curl the right armpit towards the left knee, keeping the elbows open.
   Imagine you have a golf ball under your chin so you do not pull the head forward and strain the neck.
   Scoop the stomach.

   ii) **Breathe In**, release the torso until the shoulderblades almost touch the floor and change sides.

   iii) Roll to the other side and repeat to that side.

4. **KEY POINTS:** Keep the shoulderblades off the floor at all times.
   Keep the elbow open.
   Turn the head and shoulders and look to the side for maximum rotation of the torso
   (where the eyes go, the body follows).
   Keep the hips still, planted into the mat.
   B-Line at all times.

5. **CARE:**
   Keep the elbows open so there is less strain on the neck.
   Keep the chin off the chest, eyes forward at 45° except when turning.
   When turning to the side keep both shoulders off the floor.

6. **REPETITIONS:** One set of ten to each side.

NOTES

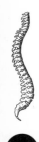

EXERCISE # 77
WRIST AND FOREARM STRENGTHENER

1. **PREREQUISITES:** Nil.

2. **PURPOSE:** To strengthen the wrists and forearms for all racquet sports and sports which require finger or wrist strength.

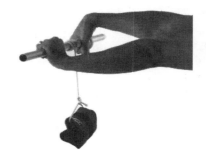

3. **EXERCISE:** Get a piece of thin rope approximately 1.5 meters long. Drill a hole through a wooden pole (30 cms long) and pass the rope through the hole and tie a knot at this end. Tie a weight or a bag of sand at the other end.

   Starting position: Stand up and **B-Lining**, hold the pole at shoulder height in front of you, arms extended. If the weight is resting on the floor, make the rope shorter.

   i) Always keeping the pole in the palm of the hand, slowly open the palm of the right hand and turn the wrist back to take a hold of the underside of the pole. Grip the pole and rotate the right wrist forward as far as possible so the knuckles are pointing towards the floor.

   ii) At the same time turn the left wrist back and take a grip of the pole. Now the left wrist extends forward as far as possible.

   iii) Keep repeating this proceedure, taking the wrist through it extreme ranges of forward and backward motion until the rope has wound all the way up the pole. There should be enough pole for the rope to roll onto without hindering the hand grip.
   Breathe normally.

   iv) Once the rope is totally rolled up, reverse the wrist movement so you unroll the weight down to the floor. Do not let the pole slide through the fingers!

   v) When the rope is unrolled, <u>do not stop</u>. Continue the unrolling action of the wrist so the rope once again begins to wind onto the pole!
   Repeat this movement up and down 4 times.

4. **KEY POINTS:** At the end of this you may feel as if the muscles in the forearm feel like bursting through the skin because they are so pumped up!
   Rotate the wrists as fully forward and backwards as possible.
   Do not let the ends of the pole swing up and down, keep it level to the floor throughout the exercise.

5. **CARE:** Vary the weight according to your requirements and strength.
   This is a challenge! Do as many wrist rolls of the rope as possible.
   This may be only up and down once to start. Aim for three times up and down!
   Adjust the weight if it becomes too easy.
   Keep the shoulders upright without hunching.
   Do not lean backwards.

   For those with weaker shoulders, this exercise can be done with the elbows by the sides and the forearms horizontal to the floor to start.

NOTES

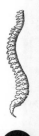

EXERCISE # 78
NECK STRETCHES

1. **PREREQUISITES:** Tight neck!

2. **PURPOSE:** To loosen tight neck muscles.

3. **EXERCISE: Starting position:**
   Sit upright on a chair or on a bench (Figure i) on your sit
   bones. Feet hip distance apart and planted on or off the floor.
   (Hold firmly onto the bench or one of the back legs of the chair,
   below seat level with the right hand).

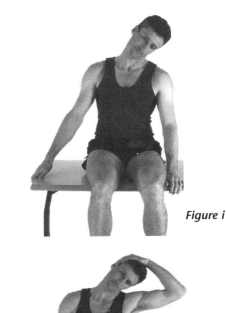

Figure i

   i) Breathe Out and stretch the left ear to the left shoulder,
   pressing both shoulders to the floor. This stretch should
   be felt strongly on the right side of the neck.

   ii) Breathe Out and as the neck stretches to the side, slightly
   turn the head to the ceiling. This stretch should be felt slightly
   to the front of the neck.

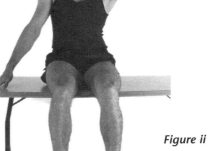

   iii) Breathe Out and as the neck stretches to the side, slightly
   turn the head to the floor. This stretch should be felt slightly
   to the back of the neck.

4. **KEY POINTS:** The stretch should be mild to start.
   Continue only if the feeling of the stretch is a **good** stretch.

Figure ii

5. **CARE:** If there is any discomfort in the neck, stop the exercise.

6. **REPETITIONS:** The above stretches are done to 6 -10 Breaths in and out to each side of the head.

ADVANCED:
   A stronger stretch can be obtained by placing the opposite hand on the top of the head and slightly
   towards the ear of the side being stretched (Figure ii).

   On the **Breathe Out**, press the head up against the pressure of the hand without the head moving.
   This isometric stretch will allow the neck muscles to lengthen further. Do not pull the head to the floor!

   Breathe In and allow the head to relax further before repeating.
   Press the shoulder, on the side being stretched, firmly to the floor.
   The resistance from the hand on the head should be no more than 50% to start.

NOTES

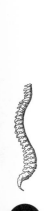

EXERCISE # 79
SEATED SPINE ROTATION

1. **PREREQUISITES:** Side to side (#23), corkscrew (#47-II) or pendulum (#62).

2. **PURPOSE:** To stretch the tight muscles of the spine and obliques to increase rotational mobility.

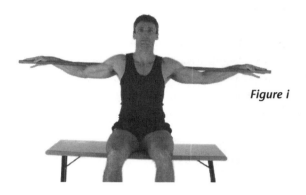

Figure i

3. **EXERCISE: Starting position:**
   Sit upright on a chair or on a bench (Figure i) on your sit bones. Feet hip distance apart and planted on the floor. Place a long pole across the back of the shoulders horizontal to the floor, arms lengthened along the pole with the hands holding onto the top of it.

   i) B-Line, **Breathe Out** and stretch the left shoulder to a point behind you, keeping the arms horizontal and pressing both shoulders to the floor.

   ii) Breathe In as the torso returns to the central position.

   iii) Repeat to the other side.

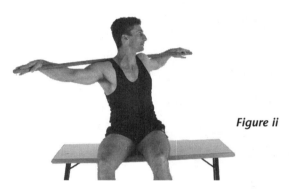

Figure ii

4. **KEY POINTS:** The stretch should be mild to start. Only if the feeling of the stretch is a **good** stretch, continue. Turn the head around as much as you can - where the eyes go, the body follows! Keep the pole horizontal to the floor at all times. Keep the shoulder blades pressed to the hips. Keep the hips square at all times.

5. **CARE:** If there is any discomfort in the back, shoulders or neck, stop the exercise.

6. **REPETITIONS:** Ten to each side. Once proficient with this exercise, the movement can be speeded up.

NOTES

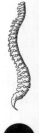

EXERCISE # 80
CUSHION SQUEEZE

1. **PREREQUISITES:** Nil.

2. **PURPOSE:** To strengthen and tone the inner thighs (adductors).

3. **EXERCISE: Starting position:**
   Lie on your back on the floor with the knees bent
   and a firm cushion or several pillows placed between
   the knees. The feet should be flat on the floor about
   30cms apart.

   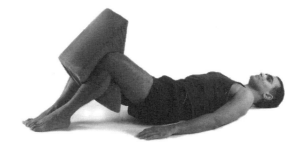

   i) B-Line, **Breathe Out** as you squeeze the cushion
   without tilting the pelvis or squeezing the buttocks.

   ii) Breathe In as you release ONLY 10% of the squeeze before repeating.

4. **KEY POINTS:** The squeeze should be mild to start.
   Gradually keep squeezing harder.
   To make the exercise even more effective, turn the toes in (pigeon toed) and feel the difference!
   THIS EXERCISE CAN ALSO BE DONE WITH ABDOMINAL CURLS! Curl up on the squeeze.

5. **CARE:** If there is any discomfort in the groin - stop. This exercise should only be felt in the inner thighs
   and not in the muscle attachments.

6. **REPETITIONS:** Two sets of ten squeezes, 15 second rest between each set.

NOTES

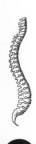

ISOTONER™ ROUTINES

The following series of exercises is done with an IsoToner™ or length of Theraband or similar wide elastic. The IsoToner™ is particularly useful as it comes with a handle and cork balls for a better grip, as well as a piece of rope for locking into a door or tying to a door handle. (Please see the end of this book for instructions on purchasing an IsoToner™). There are no prerequisite exercises for this series and anyone should be able to manage the exercises comfortably. As the IsoToner™ comes in various strengths, there is a suitable resistance for everyone.

The photographs are straightforward and clearly describe the movements required. All repetitions are one to two sets of ten repetitions per side.

CAUTION: NEVER PULL THE IsoToner™ DIRECTLY INTO YOUR FACE.

EXERCISE # IT 1
POINTING THE FOOT (PLANTAR FLEXION)

This exercise strengthens the calf muscles, the intrinsic muscles of the foot and the ankle joint.
Make sure that the toe is pointed in line with the knee.
Using the muscles of the feet press through the ball of the toe, stretching the top of the foot.
These muscles are necessary for jumping, rising onto the ball of the foot and balancing on the ball of the foot.

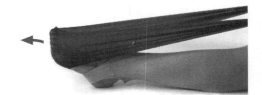

EXERCISE # IT 2
POINTING THE TOES

Strengthens the smaller muscles and tendons in the bottom of the foot. These are important for strengthening the toes. After the foot has extended through the ball of the foot, work only on flexion and extension of the toes, without flexing the foot at the ankle. Do not crunch the toes when extending. For dancers, this is necessary for pointe work, jumping and developing a pleasing line of the foot.

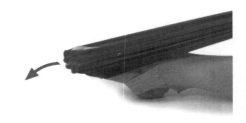

EXERCISE # IT 3
DORSI FLEXION OF THE ANKLE

Support the working foot by resting it on the bent knee.
Keep the foot pointed and apply pressure from the IsoToner™.
Draw the foot towards the knee working the muscles and tendon on the top of the foot. This strengthens the front of the ankle and the muscles on the outside (lateral side) of the calf to provide ankle support.
Dorsi flexion is necessary when landing from a jump.

EXERCISE # IT 4
EVERSION OF THE ANKLE

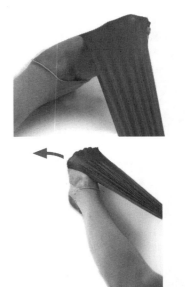

This strengthens the muscles surrounding the ankle and the muscles on the lateral side (outside) of the calf, by working on straightening the foot from a turned in or inverted position. This strengthening will help prevent ankle sprains and help in their speedy recovery. It also helps with stabilizing the ankle joint on flat surfaces or when rising onto the toe. For dancers, this strength is important in preventing 'sickling' of the foot.

EXERCISE # IT 5
INVERSION OF THE METATARSAL JOINT

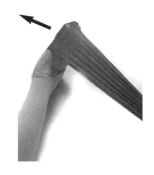

This will develop muscles in the front (anterior) part of the lower leg along the shin bone. This is necessary in stabilizing the muscles of the ankle and will help prevent rolling of the foot.

EXERCISE # IT 6
ADDUCTION OF THE INNER THIGH

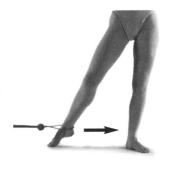

Place the rope end of the IsoToner™ in a door at calf level and close the door with the loop on the other side of the door. This will hold the IsoToner™ securely. This exercise strengthens the inner thigh muscles (adductors) of the working leg and, more importantly, the adductor muscles of the supporting leg. The leg is turned out with the IsoToner™ wrapped around the ankle, draw the heel towards the supporting foot. The muscle that is actually worked is from the top of the inner thigh.
As you release the foot, point it, keeping tension in the IsoToner™.
For dancers, this exercise develops the stability of the standing leg, helps build speed for petite allegro, and is necessary for batterie (cabrioles, entrachat six, entrachat huit, switching legs in double tours, etc.).

EXERCISE # IT 7
FLEXION AND EXTENSION OF THE LEG
WHILE USING OUTWARD ROTATION OF THE HIP JOINTS

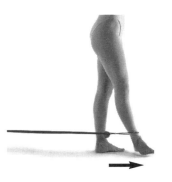

This is another exercise to strengthen the inner thigh muscles of both legs. This helps greatly with the external rotation of the thigh (femur). If there is any discomfort in the knee joint, bend the knee slightly.
Start with both legs together and extend the working foot forward as far as possible pointing the foot at the same time, then returning back to the start position.

EXERCISE # IT 8
HYPEREXTENSION TO EXTENSION

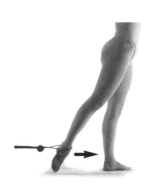

This exercise is designed to strengthen the front of the inner thigh. The resistance required to bring the leg from hyperextended (behind you) to the extended (legs together) position is helpful in working the muscles around, and especially in the front of, the hip socket.
Perform the exercise without arching the back when the leg hyperextends (B-Lining will help a great deal).

EXERCISE # IT 9
FLEXION TO EXTENSION ON THE BACK

Place the loop of the IsoToner™ over the top of a door and shut the door so the loop is securely fastened.
Lye on your back and place one foot in the handle of the IsoToner™.
Keeping both legs turned out, draw the working leg down to the floor.
This movement strengthens and tones the posterior (behind) part of the legs, including the gluteus (buttock) muscles.
This strength is required for hip placements and stability in the pelvic region (dancers: for jumps and adagios).

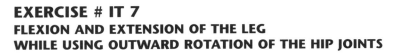

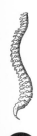

EXERCISE # IT 10
PRONE HYPEREXTENSION TO EXTENSION

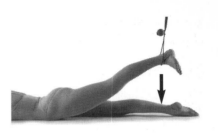

Lying on the stomach, B-Line, keep the hip bones flat on the
floor and externally rotate the legs. The resistance will
create strength and tone in the front of the thighs.

EXERCISE # IT 11
BICEPS

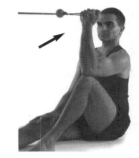

Hold the handle and sit 1 to 2 meters away.
Rest the working elbow on the bent knee.
Draw the handle to the shoulder stretching the IsoToner™.
Resist the tension upon release.
Feel as if the middle of the forearm is drawing towards the bicep,
rather than the hand towards the shoulder.

EXERCISE # IT 12
TRICEPS

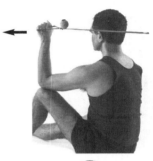

Sit on the floor with your back to the door about 1 to 1.5
meters away. Rest the working elbow on the bent knee
and extend the arm to a fully extended position.
Resist upon the release.

EXERCISE # IT 13
PECTORALS

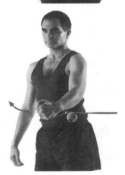

Stand sideways to a door about 1 to 2 meters away,
hold the handle and with a slightly flexed (bent)
elbow draw the IsoToner™ across the chest.
Keep the elbow in a fixed position and do not rotate
the upper body to move the arm further.

EXERCISE # IT 14
PECTORALS AND DELTOIDS

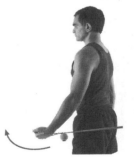

Stand with your back to the door about 1 to 2 meters away.
Hold the handle and keep the elbow in a flexed position.
Draw the handle forward to the hip and then continue forward
to shoulder level. Resist upon the return.
Keep the upper body stable.

EXERCISE # IT 15
LATISSIMUS DORSI

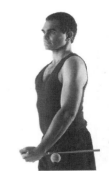
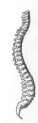

Stand sideways to the door about 1 to 2 meters away.
The arm is holding the IsoToner™ taut away from the body.
Draw the IsoToner™ to your side pressing the arm to the floor.
To better connect the lat, imagine you are squashing an orange
under the armpit as you press the arm to your side.
Resist upon the return.

EXERCISE # IT 16
BACK

Face the door about 1 to 2 meters away. With the arm extended forward at chest level, draw the handle parallel to the floor as far to the outside as possible. Keep the shoulders square to the door at all times. Imagine drawing the shoulder blades together and this will strengthen the rhomboid muscles between the shoulder blades.

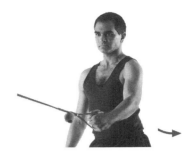

EXERCISE # IT 17
OVERHEAD

Stand sideways to the door with the working arm extended to the ceiling and about 45° to the door.
Keeping a slight bend in the elbow, extend the arm overhead away from the door. This exercise will work the shoulder muscles. If there is any discomfort in the neck, stop the exercise.

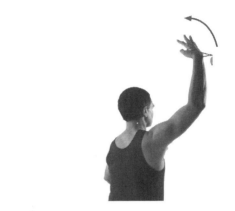

EXERCISE # IT 18
SIDE STRETCH

Standing sideways to the door with the IsoToner™ secured at the bottom of the door, place the free hand on the side of the head keeping the elbow open wide. Stretch to the side, extending through the tip of the elbow in an arc so the side does not crunch - lift up and out of the hip as if stretching over a ball.
Keep the hips firm and square. This is an important exercise for strengthening the side muscles (quadratus lumborum).

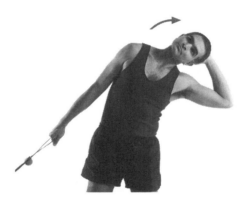

NOTES

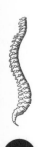

"Physical fitness can neither be acquired by wishful thinking nor by outright purchase. However, it can be gained through performing these (daily) exercises conceived for this purpose by the founder of Contrology® whose unique methods accomplish this desirable result by successfully counteracting the harmful, inherent conditions associated with modern civilization."
- Return To Life Through Contrology®

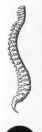

CHAPTER 6

MOVE YOURSELF OUT OF PAIN

Many people who are in pain and have passed the acute stage of their problem are still reluctant to move the body into the areas where the pain previously existed. This protective attitude of the body can be detrimental in the long term to the well-being of the individual. They have built up a fear of what was once a normal movement and has now become an 'excessive' one.

This mental protection of the physical structure inhibits recovery, rehabilitation and progress to normal movement. In the long term, an imbalance is created, which the body will accept as normal and the mind, eventually, also accepts.

Case Study

A middle aged man of slightly larger than normal build had dislocated his right shoulder 8 times in the previous 2 years. Previous rehabilitation exercises to that point involved raising weights, in a standing position, up to shoulder level and no higher.

When queried about the mobility of the joint, the patient responded that he was only able to raise the arm to shoulder height and would not attempt to raise it any higher (possibly, for fear of another dislocation) even if no weight was involved.

The last dislocation had occurred 8 months previously; the patient was convinced that his current range of movement was set for all time.

After a series of arm weights while lying supine on a narrow bench (nothing above shoulder height), the client was then told to lie face down. He was asked to raise the arms out to the sides to bench level and return to the start position. This was well within the client's perceived comfort zone and several repititions were easily completed.

After several of these movements, the client was then asked to raise the left arm to the left ear and the right arm to the right hip - and then alternate the movement (similar to a marching movement). This was accomplished without any effort or fear. When the right arm was raised to the ear on the third occasion the client was asked to hold the position and to imagine that he was in an upright position. This came as quite a surprise to the client as the arm was above head height. He was then asked to stand and repeat the movement without fear. Once this fear had been overcome the rehabilitation of the shoulder was more effective, with faster results.

The ultimate goal of any therapeutic or rehabilitation exercise program is to achieve pain free movement.

Here we shall discuss general rehabilitation exercises for the various parts of the body, in cases where the condition is no longer in the acute phases and the treating practitioner has given the clearance for a post-acute exercise program.

It is important to realize that the commencement of an exercise program does not mean immediate relief. Even though the benefits may be immediate, it is a case of the mind being willing (to achieve a normal lifestyle), but the body is still physically weak.

Too often has it been reported that when the symptoms of pain have 'disappeared' for some minutes, the patient assumes that the condition is fixed and he is able to return to normal activity. Sadly, this is far from the truth. The feeling of wellbeing may only be temporary. Although the injury may have taken only a matter of seconds to inflict, it may take months to repair. This may be very frustrating to the individual who is on a mission to be better in the shortest time possible. Remember, it was the tortoise who won the race!

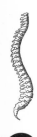

The exercise rehabilitation process has two main objectives in order to return the patient to normal activity:

1) First, to reduce the recovery time for each episode when the injured area is affected by over exersion, either intentional or accidental.

2) Secondly, to substantially strengthen the area.

What is meant by **1)** above is say, for example, an individual has lower back pain. They have not begun any exercise program, however, when their back 'goes out' it takes two days for the pain to diminish. The implementation of a personalized exercise program does not mean the problem is solved overnight. If the back again 'goes out' the program, if effectively implemented, should reduce the recovery time, previously 2 days, to less than that, possibly by only a few hours, and each time less still. As muscular stability is achieved, this should continue to reduce.

There may be setbacks along the way where more pain may be experienced. A reason for this being that, as the program progresses, the imbalance already accentuated in the individual because of the injury, is exacerbated. This is owing to the fact that the stronger muscles continue to dominate the movement. The weaker muscles tend initially to lag behind. This produces further imbalances as the strong muscles 'pull' the structure out of alignment. This is usually indicated by the fact that discomfort occurs and remains no matter what stretches are prescribed to alleviate the discomfort. This discomfort is easily remedied by gentle manipulation to 'realign' the problem area and the program can recommence. (Please consult your manipulative therapist if this occurs.)

When attending these 'realignment' sessions with a qualified practitioner, it is important to remember that no exercises should be done for at least 24-36 hours after the treatment in order for it to 'settle' into the muscular system.

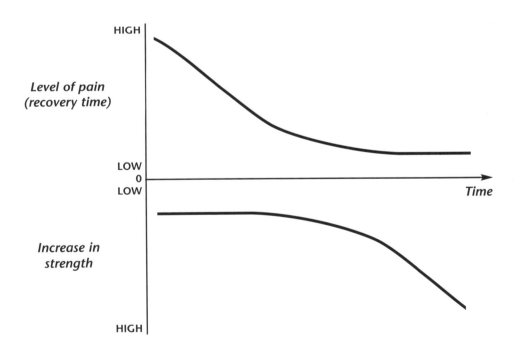

As the recovery time approaches zero, the true strengthening phase of the program can begin. Keep in mind the guidelines mentioned in Chapter III - Joint Strain.

THE CONDITIONS AND THE EXERCISES WHICH BRING RELIEF

In the descriptions of the conditions listed below, the exercises have been numbered to assist in quick reference for that condition. If the exercise is new, a description is included.

THE ANKLES AND FEET

For weak ankles and feet, including pronation, supination, flat feet and weak toes:

All ankle IsoToner™ work # IT 1 to IT 5

Plus
8-1, 8-2   Calf stretches

THE KNEE

For weak knee joints including chondromalacia of the patella and patella tracking syndrome:

8-1, 8-2   Calf stretches
26   Ankle weights

Plus IsoToner™:
IT 6   standing adduction
IT 8   hip extension
IT 7   hip flexion

THE HIP JOINT

IsoToner™ work # IT 6 to IT 10

Plus
70   HUNDREDS - HELICOPTER
20   SINGLE LEG STRETCH
22   SINGLE LEG CIRCLES WITH ANKLE WEIGHTS
62   PENDULUM
49   SIDE KICK I
56   SIDE KICK II
26   ANKLE WEIGHTS
72   SIDE STRETCHES

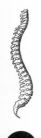

THE BACK

Lower back pain is one of the most common complaints in western society. The complaints range from minor back ache, which can be fixed with massage, manipulation or anti-inflammatories, to more serious cases. Cases such as disc protrusions, spondylolisthesis (the forward slippage of one vertebra on another), to those that require surgery.

Clearly graduated exercise programs are the best long term management for low back pain. This takes the form of gradual stretching and strengthening.

It is often more important to know what NOT to do, as these movements are the ones that can regress the program and irritate the condition.

Listed are some of the movements to avoid for certain conditions, followed by simple routines to practice. For all back problems the start stretches, hamstrings and quadricep stretches are to be completed unless there are contra-indications to the stretches.

The next three stretches are to be completed in all cases unless indications are that they are actually impossible to achieve even in the mildest form.

# 3 to 6	START STRETCHES
# 9	Appropriate Hamstring Stretch
# 11 to 13	Quadriceps stretches (Lying, standing or kneeling, depending on the tightness of the quadriceps).

For **posterior disc bulges** avoid any forward flexion exercises.
Follow Exercises:

# 24	STOMACH STRETCH
# 25	ABDOMINAL CURLS
# 20	SINGLE LEG STRETCH (with cushion)
# 21	DOUBLE LEG STRETCH (with cushion)
# 22	SINGLE LEG CIRCLES
# 18	HUNDREDS (with cushion)

For one sided **sciatic** problems, avoid exercises that contract the lower back muscles on the side where the sciatic pain is located. Stretch the tight side.
Follow the Exercises below paying particular emphasis on repeating twice as many sets on the tight side of the back:

# 7	SPIRAL STRETCH
# 44	SPINE ROTATION
# 25	PAC
# 38	SINGLE LEG STRETCH WITH OBLIQUE CURLS (TWICE AS MANY ON THE WEAK SIDE)
# 50-1	SIDE LEG LIFTS
# 21	DOUBLE LEG STRETCH
# 43	SWIMMING
# 72	SIDE STRETCH

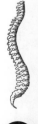

For **sciatic pain down both legs** avoid hyperextending the lower back.
Follow Exercises:

As for scoliosis on one side as well as

| # 51 | PELVIC CURL |
| # 73 | CAT STRETCH |

For **scoliosis** avoid leaning the torso to the short side of the curve.
The exercise program is the same as that for one sided sciatic pain.

For lumbar **lordosis** avoid arching the back in that area.
Follow exercises:

# 2	STANDING SPINE ROLL
# 45	SPINE STRETCH
# 18	HUNDREDS
# 32	CO-ORDINATION
# 20	SINGLE LEG STRETCH
# 21	DOUBLE LEG STRETCH
# 22	SINGLE LEG CIRCLES
# 25	CURLS
# 76	OBLIQUE CURLS
# 51	PELVIC CURLS
# 73	CAT STRETCHES
# 44	SPINE ROTATION
# 1	REST POSITION

For **cervical lordosis**, lie on the floor and place the arms at shoulder height away from the body with palms facing up. Place a small, soft cushion under the arch of the neck and, breathing out, press the neck onto the cushion, without rounding the shoulders.

Also do:

| # 78 | Neck Stretches; and |

Sitting upright, interlock the fingers behind the head. Stretch the chin to the chest and, breathing out, resist with the hands as you try to stretch the BACK of the neck to the ceiling. (Do not lift from the top of the head). Press the shoulderblades to the floor. Repeat 10 times.

SHOULDERS

For shoulder problems and kyphosis (mid/upper thoracic spine) avoid forward flexion of the back in that area.

Follow exercises:
(usually with a cushion under the forehead to support the neck in a stretched position)

# 39	STOMACH STRETCH
# 43	SWIMMING
# 30	POLE
# 28	ARM WEIGHTS
# 29	ARM SWINGS
# 78	NECK STRETCHES

The following basic routine is suggested for most low grade low back pain:

# 45	SPINE STRETCH
# 23	SIDE TO SIDE
# 18	HUNDREDS
# 32	CO-ORDINATION
# 21	DOUBLE LEG STRETCH
# 20	SINGLE LEG STRETCH
# 25	PAC
# 24	STOMACH STRETCH
# 51	PELVIC CURL
# 44	SPINE ROTATION
# 73	CAT STRETCH

As the exercises become less of a challenge, progress to the next version of the exercise, keeping in mind all the finer points of the exercise listed under Key Points and Care Notes.

THE CHALLENGE

In order to progress from the basic routine a list of exercises in progressive order has been compiled. If you are unable to complete one of the exercise perfectly in that group, you should not attempt to proceed to the next stage until that routine is achieved correctly.

The challenge is to control the manner in which the routine is performed, not how many can be achieved in the shortest period of time.

The basic routine is adequate for all levels of beginners of any age, including children (if your child is experiencing a growth spurt, first check with your medical practitioner or a qualified Pilates Practitioner).

Although the Pilates Method has become widely known for its association with rehabilitation of many types of injuries and conditions, the Challenge routines described here do not take injuries or unusual conditions into account. Therefore, they should not be attempted without first consulting a qualified Pilates Practitioner.

For the convenience of those wishing to record their progress during the various stages of the programs, we have included charts covering 7 levels of the Pilates Method.
Complete one stage at a time. Do the exercises three times a week (more if you wish). In the box for that exercise and date, state the level of effort or challenge you felt for the exercise e.g. chart below shows on Monday the standing spine roll was an effort of 7 out of 10.
If the challenge falls below 5 out of 10 on the effort scale, then progress to a harder version of the exercise.
If there isn't a harder version, then progress to a different but similar exercise which poses a challenge.
When 75% of the exercises in that stage are completed with ease, move on to the next stage, but regularly go back to the exercises you found a challenge until you are comfortable with them. Photocopy the charts to add further weeks to the program, if you wish.

Good luck! You will be glad you took the opportunity and I am pleased to have been able to present you the possibility to change your life in some positive way.

PILATES INSTITUTE OF AUSTRALASIA

EXERCISE	WEEK 1				WEEK 2				WEEK 3		
PROGRAM DATE 9-9-99	M	W	F		M	W	F		M	W	F
#2 STANDING SPINE ROLL	7	6	4								
#3 to 7 START STRETCHES	7	6	7								
#9-1 HAMSTRING STRETCH	8	8	7								
#12 QUAD STRETCH	9	8	7								
#45 SPINE STRETCH	7	7	6								
#50-I SIDE LEG LIFTS I	8	8	7								
#16 PREPARATION	8	7	6								
#18 HUNDREDS	8	8	8								
#32 CO-ORDINATION	8	7	8								
#20 SINGLE LEG STRETCH	6	6	6								
#21 DOUBLE LEG STRETCH	8	7	8								
#25 PAC	8	8	8								
#73 CAT STRETCH	6	6	6								
#28-1 ARM WEIGHTS	8	7	7								
#29 ARM SWINGS I	6	6									
#1 REST POSITION											

BASIC ROUTINE

# 2	STANDING SPINE ROLL
# 3 to 7	START STRETCHES
# 9-I	HAMSTRING STRETCH
# 12	QUAD STRETCH
# 45	SPINE STRETCH
# 50-I	SIDE LEG LIFTS I
# 16	PREPARATION
# 18	HUNDREDS
# 32	CO-ORDINATION
# 20	SINGLE LEG STRETCH
# 21	DOUBLE LEG STRETCH
# 25	PAC
# 73	CAT STRETCH
# 28-1	ARM WEIGHTS
# 29	ARM SWINGS-I
# 1	REST POSITION

STAGE I

# 2	STANDING SPINE ROLL
# 3 to 7	START STRETCHES
# 10	HAMSTRING
# 13	QUAD STRETCH
# 45	SPINE STRETCH
# 44	SPINE ROTATION
# 48	SAW
# 16	PREPARATION
# 19	HUNDREDS
# 25	PAC
# 76	OBLIQUE CRUNCHES
# 20	SINGLE LEG STRETCH
# 21	DOUBLE LEG STRETCH
# 33	ROLL-UP
# 37	ROLLING
# 47-I	CORKSCREW
# 24	STOMACH STRETCH
# 28-I/II	ARM WEIGHT II
# 26-I/II	ANKLE WEIGHTS
# 29-I/II	ARM SWINGS
# 30	POLE

STAGE II

# 3 to 7	START STRETCHES
# 9-2	HAMSTRINGS
# 13	QUADS KNEELING
# 76	OBLIQUE CURLS
# 23	SIDE TO SIDE
# 31	HUNDREDS
# 47-II	CORKSCREW II
# 62	PENDULUM
# 33	ROLL-UP
# 46	OPEN LEG ROCKER
# 20	SINGLE LEG STRETCH
# 36-I	DOUBLE LEG STRETCH
# 43	SWIMMING
# 49	SIDE KICK
# 28	ARM WEIGHTS
# 29	ARM SWINGS
# 30	POLE
# 72	SIDE STRETCH

STAGE III

# 3 to 7	START STRETCHES
# 9-2	HAMSTRINGS (LADDER)
# 13	QUADS KNEELING
# 23	SIDE TO SIDE
# 47-II	CORKSCREW II
# 62	PENDULUM
# 63	NECK PULL
# 76	OBLIQUE CRUNCHES
# 38	SINGLE LEG STRETCH WITH TWIST
# 60	HUNDREDS
# 36-II	DOUBLE LEG STRETCH
# 60/61	ROLL-OVER
# 69	HIP CIRCLES
# 64	JACKNIFE
# 58	SEAL
# 53-1	TEASER
# 40	SINGLE LEG KICK
# 28	ARM WEIGHTS
# 29	ARM SWINGS
# 72	SIDE STRETCH
# 30	POLE

STAGE IV

# 3 to 7	START STRETCHES
# 9-2	HAMSTRINGS
# 13	QUADS LUNGE
# 31	HUNDREDS
# 25	PAC
# 76	OBLIQUE CURLS
# 63	NECK PULL
# 20	SINGLE LEG STRETCH
# 36-II	DOUBLE LEG STRETCH-II
# 47-II	CORKSCREW II
# 46	OPEN LEG ROCKER
# 34	ROLL-OVER
# 61	ROLL-OVER BENT LEGS
# 53-I	TEASER I
# 54	LEG PULL FRONT
# 55	LEG PULL BACK
# 64	JACKNIFE
# 59	CONTROL BALANCE
# 28	ARM WEIGHTS
# 26-1	ANKLE WEIGHTS CIRCLES
# 29-I/II	ARM SWINGS
# 30	POLE
# 72	SIDE STRETCH

STAGE V

# 3 to 7	START STRETCHES
# 9-2	HAMSTRINGS
# 13	QUADS LUNGE
# 60	HUNDREDS
# 25	PAC
# 76	OBLIQUE CURLS
# 63	NECK PULL
# 36-III	DOUBLE LEG STRETCH - III
# 38	SINGLE LEG STRETCH WITH TWIST
# 47-III	CORKSCREW III
# 62	PENDULUM
# 69	HIP CIRCLES
# 61	ROLL-OVER BENT LEGS
# 53-II	TEASER II
# 58	SEAL
# 42-I	SWAN
# 68-I	CAN CAN EXTENSION
# 59	CONTROL BALANCE
# 65	SCISSORS
# 74	ROCKING
# 49	SIDE KICK I
# 28	ARM WEIGHTS
# 27	ANKLE WEIGHTS PRONE
# 29 I/II	ARM SWINGS
# 72-I	STANDING SIDE STRETCH

STAGE VI

# 3 to 7	START STRETCHES
# 8-2	ALTERNATING CALF STRETCH
# 10	HAMSTRINGS AT HIGH LEVEL
# 13	QUADS WITH LUNGE
# 33	ROLL UP
# 25	PAC
# 35	SINGLE LEG CIRCLE
# 38	SINGLE LEG STRETCH WITH TWIST
# 36-3	DOUBLE LEG STRETCH - EXPANSION
# 34	ROLL OVER
# 61	ROLL OVER BENT LEGS
# 44	SPINE ROTATION
# 48	SAW
# 47-III	CORKSCREW III
# 42-II	SWAN II
# 53-III	TEASER III
# 65	SCISSORS
# 66	BICYCLE
# 1	REST POSITION
# 54	LEG PULL FRONT
# 55	LEG PULL BACK
# 56	SIDE KICK II
# 57	BOOMERANG
# 59	CONTROL BALANCE
# 75-I	TWIST I
# 28-IV	ARM WEIGHTS 1-4
# 72	SIDE STRETCH
# 71	LYING SIDE STRETCH
# 29-I/II	ARM SWINGS
# 30	POLE

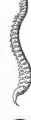

CONCLUSION

When putting the Pilates Method to work you will undoubtedly notice results within a short period of time. To achieve the most from the program, it is also important to be aware of the response your body and muscles are feeding back to you. When you feel you have mastered a program adequately, remain with that program for a further week to consolidate the connection of the mind and the body on those movements.

This may be akin to watching a film for the second time and noticing small, but important, aspects that you were unaware of the first time. If one small aspect of the film were missing, it would not dramatically change the overall message or content of the film. However, if a large section or the total of these small parts were missing, the film would give a totally different message to the viewer! You, as the viewer will gradually improve your perception and control over the smaller, once insignificant, details of the movements. As the parts fuse together to become the whole, the body will regain lost perceptions. The mind and body will work in unison and the sense of wellbeing, both mental and physical, shall produce an emotional enthusiasm that your body has not felt for some time - if ever!

So it is with the Pilates Method. I have attempted to be as precise as possible in all the description of the movements. Focus on each of them. As you become more proficient at the routines, review them after a month, even when you have progressed to the next level. Scrutinize the procedure to see if you have incorporated every aspect into the movement so that your mind and body is getting the full, clear message.

As the viewer, not only will you **see** the benefits of what the Pilates Method can do for your body, you will become so **involved** in the film that you will also **feel** the reality from deep within.

The Studios

Beyond the floor routines there are the studio-based programs. It is always advisable to check that the studio you wish to attend is a registered, certified studio with an established reputation. (Please check the internet on www.pilates.net for the studio nearest you). The studio programs are by appointment and are able to give you the full benefit of all Joe Pilates' work. Under the watchful eye of an instructor you will be guided through programs suited to your strengths and weaknesses.

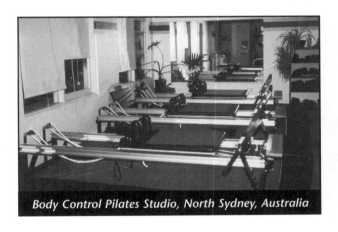
Body Control Pilates Studio, North Sydney, Australia

Within the studio environment there are a variety of pieces of equipment with curious names such as the Universal Reformer®, the Cadillac, the Wunda Chair, the Pedi-Pul and others. The use of specialised equipment challenges your body to a different level. This is not to diminish the importance of the floor routines. As a stand-alone program the floor routines can be done in any place at any time - a considerable advantage over the equipment based routines.

References

Arheim, Daniel: Modern Principles of Athletic Training. Times Mirror.

Howse, J. & Hancock, S: Dance Technique and Injury Prevention. A&C Black 1998.

Peterson, L. & Renstrom, P: Sports Injuries. Methuen.

Eisen, G. & Freidman, R: The Pilates Method of Mental and Physical Conditioning. Warner Bros.

Winter Griffith, H: Sports Injuries. The Body Press.

Kendall, F.P. & McCreary, E.K: Muscles Testing and Function. Williams & Wilkins.

Fitt, S.S: Dance Kinesiology. Schirmer Books.

Kisner, C. & Colby, L.A: Therapeutic Exercise. F.A. Davis 1988.

Kapandji, I.A: The Physiology of the Joints. Churchill Livingston.

Pilates, J: Return to Life Through Contrology.

King, B: Rules of the Bones.

Ryan, A.J. & Stephens, R.E: Dance Medicine. Pluribus Press Inc. 1987.

The Body Control Pilates Studios

<u>Australia</u>

Sydney City (Head Office)	636 George Street Sydney NSW 2000 Tel +612 9267 8223 Fax +612 9267 8226	Bondi Junction	116a Bronte Road Bondi Junction NSW 2022 Tel +612 9369 3311
North Sydney	9 Napier Street North Sydney NSW 2060 Tel +612 9929 9966	Parramatta*	181 Church Street Parramatta NSW 2150 Tel/Fax +612 9806 0179

<u>New Zealand</u>

Wellington*	142-148 Willis Street Wellington NZ Tel +64 384 1034 Fax +64 384 1036

* Independantly owned and operated licenses

For enquiries on franchises, equipment, training or registering your studio on the internet, please contact:

The Pilates Institute of Australasia
PO Box 1046
North Sydney NSW 2059
Australia

Tel +612 9267 8223
Fax +612 9267 8226

Internet: www.pilates.net

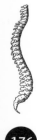

PILATES INSTITUTE OF AUSTRALASIA - BASIC ROUTINE EXERCISE CHART

EXERCISE	WEEK 1			WEEK 2			WEEK 3			WEEK 4			WEEK 5			WEEK 6			WEEK 7		
PROGRAM DATE: / /	M	W	F	M	W	F	M	W	F	M	W	F	M	W	F	M	W	F	M	W	F
#2 STANDING SPINE ROLL																					
#3 to 7 START STRETCHES																					
#9-1 HAMSTRING STRETCH																					
#12 QUAD STRETCH																					
#45 SPINE STRETCH																					
#50-1 SIDE LEG LIFTS I																					
#16 PREPARATION																					
#18 HUNDREDS																					
#32 CO-ORDINATION																					
#20 SINGLE LEG STRETCH																					
#21 DOUBLE LEG STRETCH																					
#25 PAC																					
#73 CAT STRETCH																					
#28-1 ARM WEIGHTS																					
#29 ARM SWINGS I																					
#1 REST POSITION																					

PILATES INSTITUTE OF AUSTRALASIA - STAGE I EXERCISE CHART

EXERCISE	WEEK 1			WEEK 2			WEEK 3			WEEK 4			WEEK 5			WEEK 6			WEEK 7		
PROGRAM DATE: / /	M	W	F	M	W	F	M	W	F	M	W	F	M	W	F	M	W	F	M	W	F
#2 STANDING SPINE ROLL																					
#3 to 7 START STRETCHES																					
#10 HAMSTRING																					
#13 QUAD STRETCH																					
#45 SPINE STRETCH																					
#44 SPINE ROTATION																					
#48 SAW																					
#16 PREPARATION																					
#19 HUNDREDS																					
#25 PAC																					
#76 OBLIQUE CRUNCHES																					
#20 SINGLE LEG STRETCH																					
#21 DOUBLE LEG STRETCH																					
#33 ROLL-UP																					
#37 ROLLING																					
#47-I CORKSCREW																					
#24 STOMACH STRETCH																					
#28-I/II ARM WEIGHT II																					
#26-I/II ANKLE WEIGHTS																					
#29-I/II ARM SWINGS																					
#30 POLE																					

PILATES INSTITUTE OF AUSTRALASIA - STAGE II EXERCISE CHART

EXERCISE	WEEK 1			WEEK 2			WEEK 3			WEEK 4			WEEK 5			WEEK 6			WEEK 7		
PROGRAM DATE: / /	M	W	F	M	W	F	M	W	F	M	W	F	M	W	F	M	W	F	M	W	F
#3 to 7 START STRETCHES																					
#9-2 HAMSTRINGS																					
#13 QUADS KNEELING																					
#76 OBLIQUE CURLS																					
#23 SIDE TO SIDE																					
#31 HUNDREDS																					
#47-II CORKSCREW II																					
#62 PENDULUM																					
#33 ROLL-UP																					
#46 OPEN LEG ROCKER																					
#20 SINGLE LEG STRETCH																					
#36-I DOUBLE LEG STRETCH																					
#43 SWIMMING																					
#29 SIDE KICK																					
#30 POLE																					
#72 SIDE STRETCH																					

PILATES INSTITUTE OF AUSTRALASIA - STAGE III EXERCISE CHART

EXERCISE	WEEK 1			WEEK 2			WEEK 3			WEEK 4			WEEK 5			WEEK 6			WEEK 7		
PROGRAM DATE: / /	M	W	F	M	W	F	M	W	F	M	W	F	M	W	F	M	W	F	M	W	F
#3 to 7 START STRETCHES																					
#9-2 HAMSTRINGS (LADDER)																					
#13 QUADS KNEELING																					
#23 SIDE TO SIDE																					
#47-II CORKSCREW																					
#62 PENDULUM																					
#63 NECK PULL																					
#76 OBLIQUE CRUNCHES																					
#38 SINGLE LEG STRETCH - TWIST																					
#60 HUNDREDS																					
#36-II DOUBLE LEG STRETCH																					
#60/61 ROLL-OVER																					
#69 HIP CIRCLES																					
#64 JACKNIFE																					
#58 SEAL																					
#53-I TEASER																					
#40 SINGLE LEG KICK																					
#28 ARM WEIGHTS																					
#29 ARM SWINGS																					
#72 SIDE STRETCH																					
#30 POLE																					

PILATES INSTITUTE OF AUSTRALASIA - STAGE IV EXERCISE CHART

EXERCISE	WEEK 1			WEEK 2			WEEK 3			WEEK 4			WEEK 5			WEEK 6			WEEK 7		
PROGRAM DATE: / /	M	W	F	M	W	F	M	W	F	M	W	F	M	W	F	M	W	F	M	W	F
#3 to 7 START STRETCHES																					
#9-2 HAMSTRINGS																					
#13 QUADS LUNGE																					
#31 HUNDREDS																					
#25 PAC																					
#76 OBLIQUE CURLS																					
#63 NECK PULL																					
#20 SINGLE LEG STRETCH																					
#36-II DOUBLE LEG STRETCH II																					
#47-II CORKSCREW II																					
#46 OPEN LEG ROCKER																					
#34 ROLL-OVER																					
#61 ROLL-OVER BENT LEGS																					
#53-1 TEASER I																					
#54 LEG PULL FRONT																					
#55 LEG PULL BACK																					
#64 JACKNIFE																					
#59 CONTROL BALANCE																					
#28 ARM WEIGHTS																					
#26-I ANKLE WEIGHTS CIRCLES																					
#29-I/II ARM SWINGS																					
#30 POLE																					
#72 SIDE STRETCH																					

PILATES INSTITUTE OF AUSTRALASIA - STAGE V EXERCISE CHART

EXERCISE	WEEK 1			WEEK 2			WEEK 3			WEEK 4			WEEK 5			WEEK 6			WEEK 7		
PROGRAM DATE: / /	M	W	F	M	W	F	M	W	F	M	W	F	M	W	F	M	W	F	M	W	F
#3 to 7 START STRETCHES																					
#9-2 HAMSTRINGS																					
#13 QUADS LUNGE																					
#60 HUNDREDS																					
#25 PAC																					
#76 OBLIQUE CURLS																					
#63 NECK PULL																					
#36-III DOUBLE LEG STRETCH III																					
#38 SINGLE LEG STRETCH - TWIST																					
#47-III CORKSCREW III																					
#62 PENDULUM																					
#69 HIP CIRCLES																					
#61 ROLL-OVER BENT LEGS																					
#53-II TEASER II																					
#54 LEG PULL FRONT																					
#58 SEAL																					
#42-I SWAN																					
#68-I CAN CAN EXTENSION																					
#59 CONTROL BALANCE																					
#65 SCISSORS																					
#74 ROCKING																					
#49 SIDE KICK																					
#28 ARM WEIGHTS																					
#27 ANKLE WEIGHTS PRONE																					
#29-I/II ARM SWINGS																					
#72-I STANDING SIDE STRETCH																					

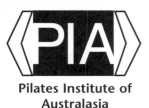

Pilates Institute of Australasia

PILATES METHOD VIDEOS

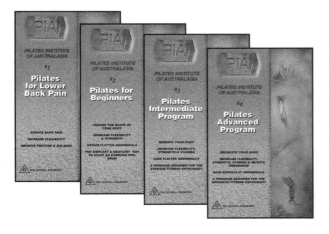

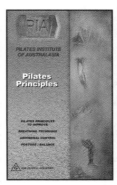

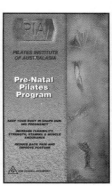

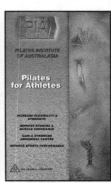

Shipping Charges (prices and shipping charges in AUS$)

ONE VIDEO ONLY:

	Air Mail	Econ. Air	Surface
Europe	$15.00	$12.00	$10.00
Asia	$11.50	$10.00	$9.00
New Zealand	$9.50	$9.00	n/a
Australia	All states - $6.60		

COMPLETE SET OF VIDEOS 1-4:

	Air Mail	Econ. Air	Surface
Europe	$31.50	$24.00	$19.00
Asia	$22.75	$19.00	$16.50
New Zealand	$17.75	$16.50	n/a
Australia	All states - $12		

Add $8 for each additional video ordered, except Australia - $5
Orders will be shipped within 10 days of availability. Please allow 2 weeks air, 3 weeks economy air and 3 months surface for delivery.

Name: _____

Postal Address: _____

Postcode: _____ State: _____ Country: _____

Telephone: _____ Fax: _____ Email: _____

Please send me...

☐ **1. Pilates for Low Back Pain** for $29.95 + p&h   ☐ **2. Pilates - Basic Floor** for $29.95 + p&h

☐ **3. Pilates - Intermediate Floor** for $29.95 + p&h   ☐ **4. Pilates - Advanced Floor** for $29.95 + p&h

OR

☐ **The complete set of videos 1-4** for only $99.95 p&h

☐ **Principles** for $29.95 + p&h   ☐ **Pre-natal** for $29.95 + p&h   ☐ **Pilates for Athletes** for $29.95 + p&h

Payment details... (For orders outside Australia, only credit card payments are accepted)

☐ Cheque ☐ Money Order   Amount: $_____   Shipping: $_____

☐ Credit Card   Amount: $_____   ☐ Bankcard   ☐ Visa   ☐ MasterCard

Card #: __ __ __ __   __ __ __ __   __ __ __ __   __ __ __ __   Expiry Date: _____/_____

Name on Card: _____

Signature on Card: _____

Send completed form plus payment to: Pilates Institute of Australasia (PIA), PO Box 1046, North Sydney NSW 2059, Australia or Fax: (+612) 9267 8226. If you have any queries call the Pilates Institute of Australasia on Tel: (+612) 9267 8223 or email: allan@pilates.net or purchase online from: www.pilates.net

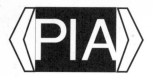

ISOTONER

The Isotoner is the ideal affordable "gym in a bag" which can help you increase your:

- *Arms and upper body*
- *Leg line*
- *Suppleness*
- *Strength*

The Isotoner is the ideal resistance aid for basic, intermediate and advanced Pilates floor routine exercises. The Isotoner is compact, affordable and easy to use.

Priced at just $29.95

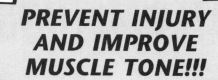

STRETCHIT!

StretchIt! is for every serious athlete who uses their ankles - thats all of you! Prevent injury and stretch your calves the easiest way with this sturdy product. Made from high grade aluminium, it can take weights up to 440lbs (200kgs), yet weighs only 2.2lbs (1kg)!

Priced at just $149

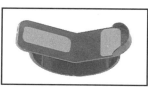

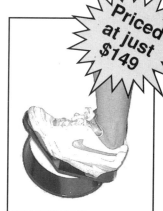

Indestructible under normal use, StretchIt! has a lifetime guarantee.

✂ -

Name: _____

Postal Address: _____

Postcode: _____ State: _____ Country: _____

Telephone: _____ Fax: _____ Email: _____

Please send me...

❏ **1 x ISOTONER** for $29.95 + $3.00 p&h ($4.50 overseas)   ❏ **2 x ISOTONER** for $49.95 + $4.50 p&h ($9.00 overseas)
NOTE: Isotoner are available in three different resistances - please indicate which: ❏ Light (green) ❏ Medium (blue) ❏ Heavy (silver)

❏ **1 x STRETCHIT!** for $149 +p&h: Europe $37.00, Asia $28.50, New Zealand $23.50, Australia $15.00

Payment details... (For orders outside Australia, only credit card payments are accepted)

❏ Cheque   ❏ Money Order   Amount: $_____

❏ Credit Card   Amount: $_____   ❏ Bankcard   ❏ Visa   ❏ MasterCard

Card #: ___ ___ ___ ___   ___ ___ ___ ___   ___ ___ ___ ___   ___ ___ ___ ___   Expiry Date: _____ /_____

Name on Card: _____

Signature on Card: _____

Send completed form plus payment to: Pilates Institute of Australasia (PIA), PO Box 1046, North Sydney NSW 2059, Australia or Fax: (+612) 9267 8226. If you have any queries call the Pilates Institute of Australasia on Tel: (+612) 9267 8223 or email: allan@pilates.net or order online: www.pilates.net